Therapeutic Recreation in the Nursing Home

by

Linda Buettner, C.T.R.S., Ph.D.

and

Shelley L. Martin

Therapeutic Recreation in the Nursing Home

by
Linda Buettner, C.T.R.S., Ph.D.
and
Shelley L. Martin

Venture Publishing, Inc.
State College, PA

Copyright © 1995
Venture Publishing, Inc.
1999 Cato Avenue
State College, PA 16801
Phone (814) 234-4561
FAX (814) 234-1651

Manuscript Editing by: Richard Yocum, Michele Barbin, Naomi Gallagher, and Katherine Young
Production by: Richard Yocum
Cover Designed and Illustrated by: Sandra Sikorski, Sikorski Design

Library of Congress Catalogue Card Number 95-60609
ISBN 0-910251-76-2

Dedication

This book is dedicated to Bonnie Godbey because she knew how to encourage, inspire, nurture, love, and live. She was a true Woman of Leisure. She could take the magic and the potential power of a moment or a friendship and expand it. She could embrace difference and sameness without feeling the need to negate the other. She taught us that we are not static souls, but always in the process of unfolding.

We love you and miss you.

Linda wishes to acknowledge . . .

Carol Kates, who assisted in transforming the work of two authors smoothly into one.

The many talented professionals at Willard Psychiatric Center who assisted in geriatric program development.

A special thanks to Suzanne Fitzsimmons, RN, and the staff and residents of the Reconstruction Home in Ithaca, NY.

My greatest debt of gratitude is to the many older adults who have taught me that one should regard life in long-term care as a time for continued growth and development and that there really is no finish line.

Shelley wishes to acknowledge . . .

The support, caring, and encouragement from Charlotte Samson.

The friendship, sharing, and support from Linda Buettner.

The support, connection, and fun shared by the "PSU Women of Leisure."

Elaine Johnson, for her gift of healing which taught me much of what I have shared in this book, and all of what I know about clinical skills and the helping relationship. I am very grateful for the time Elaine and I have worked together and for all of the wisdom and love she has shared with me.

Both authors wish to acknowledge . . .

Herberta Lundegren, Senior Associate Dean of Health and Human Development at Penn State University, for providing technical guidance for this manuscript and encouragement throughout our education and careers.

The patience of Amber Buettner, Linda's daughter, for the times she put up with us working on this book, and for the precious drawing of the pony that inspired this book.

The staff of Venture Publishing, Inc., who contributed their time and talents to the production of this text.

Table of Contents

Section Four: Evaluation

Chapter One
Introduction to Therapeutic Recreation in the Nursing Home

Activities vs. Therapeutic Recreation

Prior to 1987, the focus of recreation services in the nursing home was to provide activities that were fun and that would help the residents to pass the time of day. The purpose was clearly diversional. Popular activities included bingo, board games, birthday parties, and sing-alongs. These services were provided by the department titled "Activities" and were supervised by an Activity Director who needed no specialized training and, in most states, no more than a high school diploma. Today recreational services provided in the nursing home setting are far more diverse, are provided by therapeutic recreation departments under the direction of certified, and, in some states, licensed therapeutic recreation specialists with college training. What is the difference between activities and therapeutic recreation, and what caused the shift in focus?

The Omnibus Reconciliation Act of 1987 (OBRA '87) changed the focus of nursing home activities programs from diversional to both diversional and therapeutic. OBRA '87 states that the recreation program must meet not only the interests of the residents (diversional), but also the physical, mental, and psychosocial (therapeutic) needs of the residents. This means that the purpose of recreation is much more than just diversion, activity, or fun. The purpose of therapeutic recreation is twofold, based on the integration of the two therapeutic recreation service models: the Leisurability Model (Peterson & Gunn, 1984) and the Health and Wellness Model (Austin, 1991). The first purpose is "to facilitate the development, maintenance, and expression of an appropriate leisure lifestyle, for individuals with physical, mental, social, or emotional limitations" (Peterson & Gunn, 1984, p. 4). Second, therapeutic recreation uses "activity, recreation, and leisure to help people deal with problems that serve as barriers to health and to assist them to grow toward their highest levels of health and wellness" (Austin, 1991, p. 132). In other words, therapeutic recreation has a dual purpose of diversional and therapeutic activities.

Diversional and Therapeutic Activities

It is important to recognize that not all activities are considered therapeutic. For the purposes of this book we have broken activities down into two categories: *diversional* and *therapeutic* (see Table 1.1, page 2). Residents in our care need both types, but a recreation therapist may not need to provide the activities considered to be diversional. Aides, volunteers, and others can be trained to assist or lead diversional activities. The therapist, then, can be free to provide the assessment, planning, evaluation, and the outcome based recreation therapy sessions.

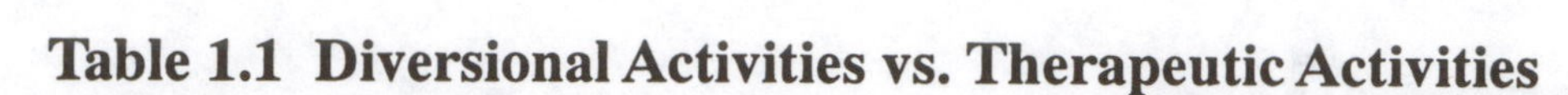

Table 1.1 Diversional Activities vs. Therapeutic Activities

Diversional Activities:	Therapeutic Activities:
-Used to entertain or divert one's thoughts from stresses of life or to fill time.	-Used to attain a specific care plan goal or objective.
-Can be lead by nontherapist or be self-guided.	-Usually guided by a therapist or highly trained professional
-Can be passive	-Often requires active involvement from the participant.
-May be large group with very little interaction between residents and peers, or residents and staff	-Done in small groups or one-to-one level, many opportunities for therapeutic interactions.
-e.g., bingo, listening to music, birthday parties	-e.g., therapeutic exercise, sensory cooking group, walking program, falls prevention exercise.

Who needs therapy instead of activities? Any resident who can not structure his or her own leisure due to a physical, mental, emotional, or social limitation will benefit from therapeutic activities.

Basic Concepts Needed for T. R. in the Nursing Home

This section provides an interpretation of the concepts of aging and leisure. Before establishing a therapeutic recreation department the staff should understand these basic concepts.

The Aging Process

AGING

The therapeutic recreation staff who work in nursing homes must not only respect and value older adults, but also become familiar with the definitions, concepts, and theories of aging. What is aging? Aging is the developmental process of growing older; it is the refinement of one's life. This process begins the day a person is born, not the day he or she retires.

An older adult has spent many years gaining unique skills, knowledge, and wisdom. Older adults are diverse in abilities and disabilities. In fact, gerontologists sometimes break old age into two categories: "young old" (65-75) and, "old old" (75+) years to help differentiate the groups.

Aging is something we all hope to do well. It brings with it many changes for the individual to cope with: social, psychological, and biological. Growing older involves changes in the individual's perceptions, social roles, functional abilities, self-concept, behavior, and approach to living. It also can mean serious changes in physical and mental health. The recreation therapist in a nursing home must understand the changes that occur due to aging and to disease. She must then provide appropriate interventions and opportunities for leisure.

THEORIES ON AGING

There is no universally accepted theory of aging. There are some biological theories, which can be divided into genetic and nongenetic theories. One of the genetic theories is the Hayflick Limit Model (1966) in which cells can only double a set number of times. His research showed that functional changes within cells are responsible for aging.

Another genetic theory is the transcription theory (Hayflick, 1983) which focuses on the first stage of genetic processing, or transcription. This theory states that with increasing age, deleterious changes occur during transcription.

Bjorksten (1974) is responsible for one of the earliest nongenetic theories of aging known as cross-linking. He looked at how large reactive protein molecules partially split, but stayed connected. In this theory molecules become cross-linked causing a loss of elasticity, sclerosis, and failure of the immune system. In other words, cross linking is responsible for the harmful effects of aging.

The free radical theory (Harmon, 1986) is based on the idea that highly charged ions whose outer orbit contains an unpaired electron cause damage at the cellular level. There is popular support for this theory, which has lead to research to inhibit free radicals. Many people now take vitamin C, selenium, and vitamin E to prevent cellular damage due to free radicals.

There are also theories of aging based in sociology. A sociologist is interested in how social roles change with maturity. For example, life begins as an infant and then proceeds developmentally to childhood, adolescence, then young adulthood. In adulthood primary social roles may change from that of a spouse or domestic partner, to parent, and grandparent. A sociologist may be interested in how the individual feels and acts when he or she becomes a grandparent for the first time.

At one point sociologists believed that aging meant a withdrawal from society and activities (Cumming & Henry, 1961). Later other sociologists theorized that aging was based on continuation and change in activity, not withdrawal from life (Havighurst, 1963). For example, an important role as independent home owner or apartment dweller changes dramatically when the individual moves into a nursing home. For some the move may be a relief after months of health problems that burdened friends and family. For others the move might seem like a devastating and sudden loss of everything meaningful. The most important thing to remember is the fact that there is vast diversity among older individuals.

Another sociological theory (Butler & Lewis, 1982; Streib, 1985) states that older people form a subculture unto themselves in which they develop their own set values, feelings, and jokes that only they can understand. This phenomenon can often be seen on a specific unit of a nursing home or in a senior housing complex.

Finally, Neugarden's Continuity Theory (1975) argues that certain tasks must be accomplished to age successfully. This theory connects biological and environmental factors, and looks at the older adult in terms of adaptation to both.

AGING ≠ DISEASE ≠ INACTIVITY

Aging does not necessarily mean illness will become a way of life. Many individuals live healthy and active lives well into their 90s. Chronic health disorders, however, are often common place in later maturity (Cockerham, 1991). Most nursing home residents have several serious health problems that cause disability. With disability, many older individuals become isolated and inactive. There is a high probability of loneliness and boredom in the resident with multiple physical health problems. The recreation therapist must be sensitive to his or her needs and limitations, and adapt activities accordingly.

Researchers estimate that 50 percent to 80 percent of nursing home residents have a diagnosable mental disorder (German et al., 1992). The majority of these residents have some form of dementia. Residents with dementia need a special approach from all staff and carefully planned recreation therapy to maintain activity levels.

The physical and mental infirmities that are often prevalent in nursing home residents frequently prevent the resident from coping with problems. The behaviors that commonly result can lead to isolation and lack of activity. It is very important that the therapist does not allow this lack of coping to turn into the lack of activity.

Leisure

Therapeutic recreation is grounded on principles of leisure. Leisure can be defined in several different ways. It can be thought of as time spent not working or doing chores. Many people think of leisure as time, calling it free time. Others think of leisure as certain specific recreational or diversional activities, such as sports, arts and crafts, or music. However, the problem with these perceptions of leisure is that they overlook the complexity of the notion of leisure. For instance, some people gain an income from their leisure interests. Would this then truly be considered leisure? What about the professional baseball player? Does he see baseball as leisure or is it his work? What about cooking, interior decorating, or do-it-yourself projects around the home? Are these activities truly leisure or are they necessary chores? Leisure is a complex concept that is difficult to define in terms of time or specific activities. There is a third way to think of leisure, and this is most helpful when leisure is to be therapeutic. Leisure can be thought of as a state of mind that results from enjoyable voluntary interaction with oneself, one's environment, or with others.

LEISURE FLOW EXPERIENCE

When a person experiences the most intense state of mind that is leisure, it is called a "flow" experience (Csikszentmihalyi, 1975). This is thought to be the optimal or "peak" leisure experience. This peak state of mind can be described as follows: first, the individual has a limited focus of attention and is totally involved in the present experience. For example, some would describe it as being "into" an activity so much that the house could fall down around them and they would not be aware of it. Second, the individual loses his or her sense of self-awareness, anxiety, and constraint. For example, some experiencing flow would not feel nervous or self-conscious while dancing in front of a crowd. He or she would also not care what others thought about them at that moment. This is like the person who is wearing a lamp shade at a party. Third, the individual loses track of time and space. He or she momentarily forgets what time it is and where he or she is. Fourth, the individual experiences enlightened perception. This means getting a great idea, understanding something totally, or seeing something in a new light. The individual might say, "oh, now I see how it all connects!" Last, the individual enjoys the experience. This is the "fun" part of leisure. It must be pleasurable or enjoyable. When all these conditions are met, an individual is said to be having a flow or peak leisure experience.

Not every leisure experience is a peak experience. Sometimes only a few of the conditions are met and sometimes none of them are met. So, the leisure state of mind can be thought of as a continuum, or a line that varies in intensity and quality. As the quality and intensity of the leisure experience increases, the individual gets closer to the peak or flow experience. The leisure state of mind is at one end of the continuum or line, and leisure lack, or nonleisure is at the other end. Nonleisure would be considered as something that is required or not done of one's own free will. See Figure 1.1.

Figure 1.1 Leisure Experience Continuum

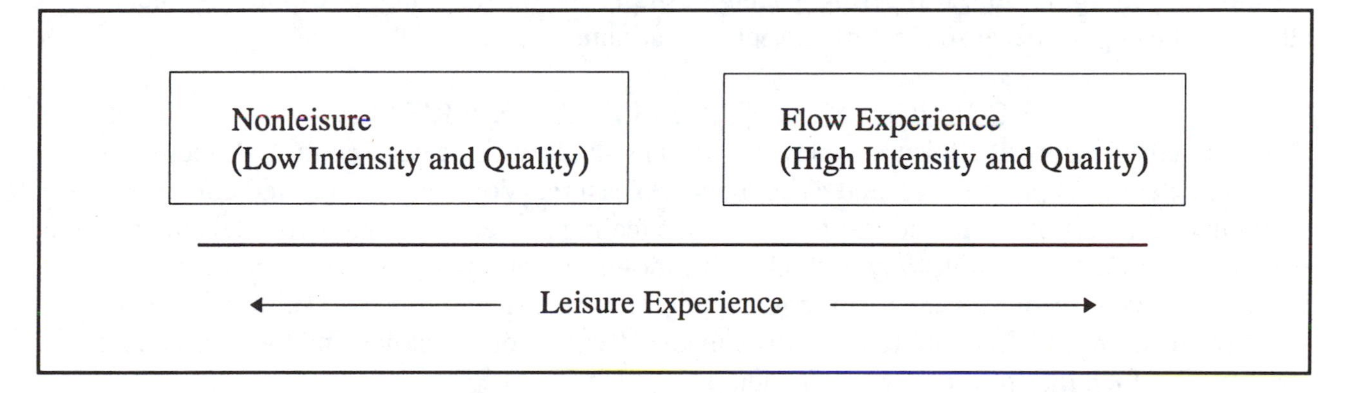

CONSTRAINTS

Constraints are barriers that keep individuals from having peak leisure experiences. Constraints are defined as anything that prevents a person from experiencing leisure. They are divided into three types: 1) intraindividual constraints, 2) extraindividual constraints, and 3) interindividual constraints (Crawford & Godbey, 1987). Constraints can be the result of illness, disability, lack of knowledge, lack of awareness, or lack of experience.

Intraindividual constraints are experienced within the resident, usually as an attitude, emotion, or thought (Crawford & Godbey, 1987). Examples of these constraints are depression, anxiety, loss of memory, disordered or impaired thinking, grief, frustration, anger, disorientation, dementia, psychosis, dependence, constraining attitudes and values, poor self-esteem, fear, and spiritual and religious beliefs. For example, someone with a diagnosis of depression would have several constraints, such as decreased attention span, lack of concentration or diminished ability to feel pleasure that would interfere with the quality and intensity of a leisure experience. These constraints would interfere with the person's ability to experience flow.

Extraindividual constraints are experienced by the individual in relationship with her or his environment or situation (Crawford & Godbey, 1987). This broad category includes physical disabilities and illness as well as situational, environmental, and historical constraints. Physical disability and illness are the constraints or barriers to leisure that are most often identified. In the nursing home these are easily found by reviewing the resident's medical chart. Some examples are amputation, paralysis, contractures, diabetes, coronary heart/artery disease, unsteady gait, decreased range of motion, vertigo, and incontinence. Sensory impairments such as vision, hearing, taste, smell, and touch are also physical constraints. Situational constraints can sometimes be found in the medical chart, such as feeding tube, oxygen use, catheter, nasogastric tube, colostomy, or nephrosotomy. The situation of being in a nursing home is also a constraint to leisure because it restricts the residents' freedom. Similarly, the use of a wheelchair, gerichair, walker, cane or other assistive devices can be constraints. This area also includes finances—lack of money to participate in desired leisure. Historical constraints are events that affect an entire community or nation, such as a war, a depression, or crisis such as a natural disaster like an earthquake, hurricane, or flood. Some of these historical constraints may make a lasting impression on an individual even though they occurred a long time ago. For instance, a strong work ethic or sense of frugality learned during the Great Depression may still constrain an individual's ability to enjoy leisure even today.

Interindividual constraints are experienced by the resident in relationship to other people (Crawford & Godbey, 1987). This category includes communication impairments, family relationships, and social relationships with friends, staff and other residents. Behavioral problems—screaming, yelling, hitting, wandering, pacing, restlessness, and refusing to respond to others are also in this category because they affect social functioning.

COMPONENTS OF A LEISURE EXPERIENCE

The main components of a leisure experience are 1) voluntary choice and control, 2) feelings of self-competence, 3) playfulness, and 4) enjoyment/pleasure. Voluntary choice and control is a very important part of the leisure experience. This feeling of freely choosing your leisure is called *perceived freedom.* A simple way to think of it is doing something by choice. According to many, perceived freedom is the main requirement for leisure (Neulinger, 1974). It includes two kinds of freedom: the freedom to participate in an activity of one's choice and the freedom from constraints which interfere with participation.

Competence is another important component of leisure. People gain an awareness of their own competence through their experience during leisure. Participants must feel they are able to participate with some degree of skill for an interaction to be satisfying. This area includes specific leisure skills such as ability to go outdoors for a walk. The main point is that the participant feels that he or she has sufficient ability to be successful in the experience.

Playfulness and enjoyment are intertwined in leisure. Certainly an activity must be enjoyable or pleasurable to be considered leisure. Linked with this is a sense of playfulness that enables the person to enjoy the activity. Playfulness also includes the willingness to take risks, to be spontaneous, and to demonstrate a sense of humor.

Leisure for Older Adults: Research Findings

Iso-Ahola (1980) has said that adults naturally decrease their leisure participation with age. Many researchers have concluded that the leisure activities of older adults are passive in nature; that is to say they are less active, solitary, and based in the home (Baley, 1955; Cowgill & Baulch, 1962; Cunningham, Montoye, Metzner & Keller, 1968; Gordon, Gaitz & Scott, 1976; Zborowski, 1962).

However, Peppers (1976) found that older adults who were social and active had a higher level of life satisfaction than those who were not. Ragheb and Griffith (1982) found that older adults with high leisure satisfaction and participation also scored high in life satisfaction. Despite the benefits of participation in leisure activities, declining physical health can be a constraint to an active leisure lifestyle for the elderly.

Baley (1955) found that "as men grow older, they like fewer recreation activities, feel indifferent towards an increasing number, and dislike an increasing number" (p. 4). If asked, most older adults are reluctant to admit that they have much leisure time (Hoar, 1961). Most of the elderly population say that their work gave them much more satisfaction than their leisure pursuits (Pfeiffer & Davis, 1971; Hooker & Ventis, 1984). The Protestant work ethic is very strong in today's elderly. They are reluctant to admit to an increase in leisure time, even in retirement, saying that most of their extra time is spent in "maintenance activities" (Bosse & Ekerdt, 1981, p. 653). Research in this area, then, must be tempered with a healthy dose of skepticism, when self-report measures are used to monitor the leisure activities of a generation that clearly does not want to admit their value. The amount of time spent in leisure time activities may be under-reported.

Several general patterns can be established in the observation of the leisure activity of older adults. Mobily (1982) postulates that the actual effect of age on adults' leisure patterns is less than the effects of socioeconomic and health status. Kelly, Steinkamp and Kelly (1986) suggest that health and physical ability regulate the activities of older adults and that their preferences tend to shift from physical to social activity as age increases. For example, National Outdoor Recreation Plans and Outdoor Recreation Resources Review Commission completed surveys of outdoor recreation participation in 1960, 1965, 1972, and 1977. They found that people over the age of 65 participated in fewer outdoor activities than younger people. Knudson (1984) found that some outdoor activities have stable participation rates over the lifespan. These are picnicking, nature walks, bird watching, and walking. McAvoy (1977) also found that the outdoor activities most frequently engaged in and enjoyed by the elderly were walking, gardening, and driving.

In a recreation participation study prepared for the Pennsylvania Department of Environmental Resources, sightseeing was found to be the most frequent outdoor activity for people age 65 and over in Pennsylvania, with 66 annual participation days per person. The next most frequent activity was jogging or walking for fitness (62 days), followed by picnicking (60 days). Bird watching and walking for fitness were the activities that held up best over the life span with participation actually increasing with age. Older adults were also found to participate in bicycling, boating, fishing, golfing, hiking, and swimming at a rate of greater than 10 days per year. We can generalize that older adults do continue to participate in outdoor activities, and that while this participation does tend to decrease as age increases, these activities still remain enjoyable and important to the older adult.

Kelly, Steinkamp and Kelly (1986) showed that participation declines in sport, exercise, and community organizations as people age. Conversely, participation in family, social, and home-based and cultural activities remain constant over the life span. Lawton, Moss and Fulcomer (1986-7) got similar results in a study of time use by older adults. The authors found that 59% of their subjects participated in interaction with family and friends. Other activities favored by most older adults include reading (54%), television viewing (85%), rest and relaxation (76%), and travel (50%).

In a study of public housing design, Nasar and Farokhpay (1985) wanted to find out how much time was spent in certain daily activities, and which of these were important to older adults in a way that would affect apartment design. The overwhelming activity of the day was television viewing (average 217 minutes per day) which was second only to sleeping (499 minutes per day). The authors also found that resting and relaxing (117 minutes per day), listening to music (181 minutes per day), looking outside (63 minutes per day), hobbies (41 minutes per day), reading and writing (69 minutes per day), and talking on the telephone (36 minutes per day) were activities of major time commitment for older adults.

Gordon, Gaitz and Scott (1976) studied leisure participation by age in the Houston area. They concluded that some activities, such as solitary activities and cooking, increased with age. Other activities, such as dancing, drinking, movies, sports, exercise, shooting, outdoor activities, travel, reading, and cultural production, decreased with age. Those activities which remained stable were found to be home-based, sedentary, inexpensive, and social in nature.

Godbey, Patterson and Szwak-Brown (1982, p. 46-48) report that retired adults engage in the following types of leisure activities: visiting others, movies, restaurants, shopping, church, walking, club meetings, education, museums, libraries, sports events, local parks, senior centers, and outdoor sports. Louis Harris and Associates (1975) polled individuals aged 65 and older as to their favorite leisure activities. They found that over 47% socialized with friends, 39% gardened, 36% both read and watched television, and 25% went for walks.

Morgan and Godbey (1978) administered the Leisure Activities Blank to 160 retired adults. Common activities that the adults had participated in prior to moving to a retirement community were: reading, driving, watching television, cooking and baking, listening to the radio, talking on the telephone, visiting friends, dining out, hiking, walking, listening to records, sewing, social drinking, watching team sports, window shopping, writing letters, sightseeing, attending concerts, movies, plays, and lectures.

In summary, many studies have identified similar activities in which older adults participate. These activities tend to be done in or around the home with family or friends. The activities tend to be a continuation of those done in the past, and are affected more by health and socioeconomic status than by age itself. Most community-based adults do not use recreational services that are available to them, and those who do tend to be more healthy and social than those who do not (Coulton & Frost, 1982).

GENDER, AGING, AND LEISURE

The aging process may affect men and women in different ways. Some say women seem to age better than men, because they live longer. However, many more women live with chronic debilitating disease. It follows that many more women than men reside in nursing homes. This is an important point because, when planning programs, the therapist must look at the needs of both women and men.

For some women leisure may be a new experience. Many women are caregivers throughout their lives. Caring for a spouse, children, aging family members leaves little time for leisure. Perhaps the only recreation the older woman had while working in the home and caregiving was to listen to the radio while she worked. A certain morning radio show may have been a very important part of her day. Maybe calling friends and family on the phone after the children were tucked in was a meaningful leisure time event. (It may have been the only time she had a few quiet minutes to herself.) Women who worked outside the home may have enjoyed going out to lunch with friends, free of the pressures of the home and work. For still other women, the church often played an important role in leisure. Family activities and obligations to others may have usurped the woman's own leisure interests. She may not have had time to develop her talents and skills.

These are all important things to consider when planning an intervention for the resident. Were there daily things that the individual enjoyed in the past? How can the recreation therapist now provide access to those important activities? For example, for years Mrs. Jones has enjoyed a morning radio show that is now scheduled during the time she is to receive her morning bath. What can the unit recreation therapist do to remove this constraint to leisure?

In the past it was more acceptable for men than women to take time for leisure. Men's leisure interests, therefore, may have developed over the years. Time to read the paper, watch the news, play cards, bowl, or hunt/fish may have been a vital part of the male's routine. The male resident may enjoy sports, cooking, handiwork, or cars. He may know his interests and have the skills he needs to participate in activities, or he too may need a refresher course. Often older men have a difficult time making social friendships. Putting together some men's groups and facilitating friendships may be one of the therapist's most important roles.

Leisure education should be included for both men and women in all long term care facilities. Educational sessions on a variety of topics should be included in the yearly plan with plenty of consideration for the wishes of the residents.

Goals of Therapeutic Recreation

One of the main goals of therapeutic recreation in the nursing home is to enable residents to have active, engaging leisure experiences. During this experience, leisure is mostly therapeutic and beneficial to the physical health and psychological growth of the participant. The role of the recreation therapist is to discover what constraints are preventing the resident from experiencing meaningful leisure, and then to develop a plan that will reduce, eliminate, or bypass those constraints. During this process, leisure experiences are developed that will increase feelings of competence, control, playfulness, and enjoyment. In this way, the leisure experience can help to meet the physical, mental, emotional, and social needs of the participant.

The Therapeutic Recreation Process

The method by which the goals of therapeutic recreation are accomplished is known as the therapeutic recreation process (Austin, 1991). This process has four distinct parts. First, a thorough assessment is completed to determine the resident's functioning levels across the many components of leisure. Second, in the planning phase, a goal plan is created for each resident. This goal plan is based on the individual needs of each resident. Third, the plan is carried out in an implementation phase. Last, in the evaluation phase, the outcomes are weighed, and the whole process begins again. The parts of the therapeutic recreation process are easy to remember if one uses the first letter of each to spell APIE as follows:

A-ssessment
P-lanning
I-mplementation
E-valuation

In the chapters that follow, each part of the therapeutic recreation process will be explained and explored as it is applied in the specific setting of the nursing home.

Section One

Assessment

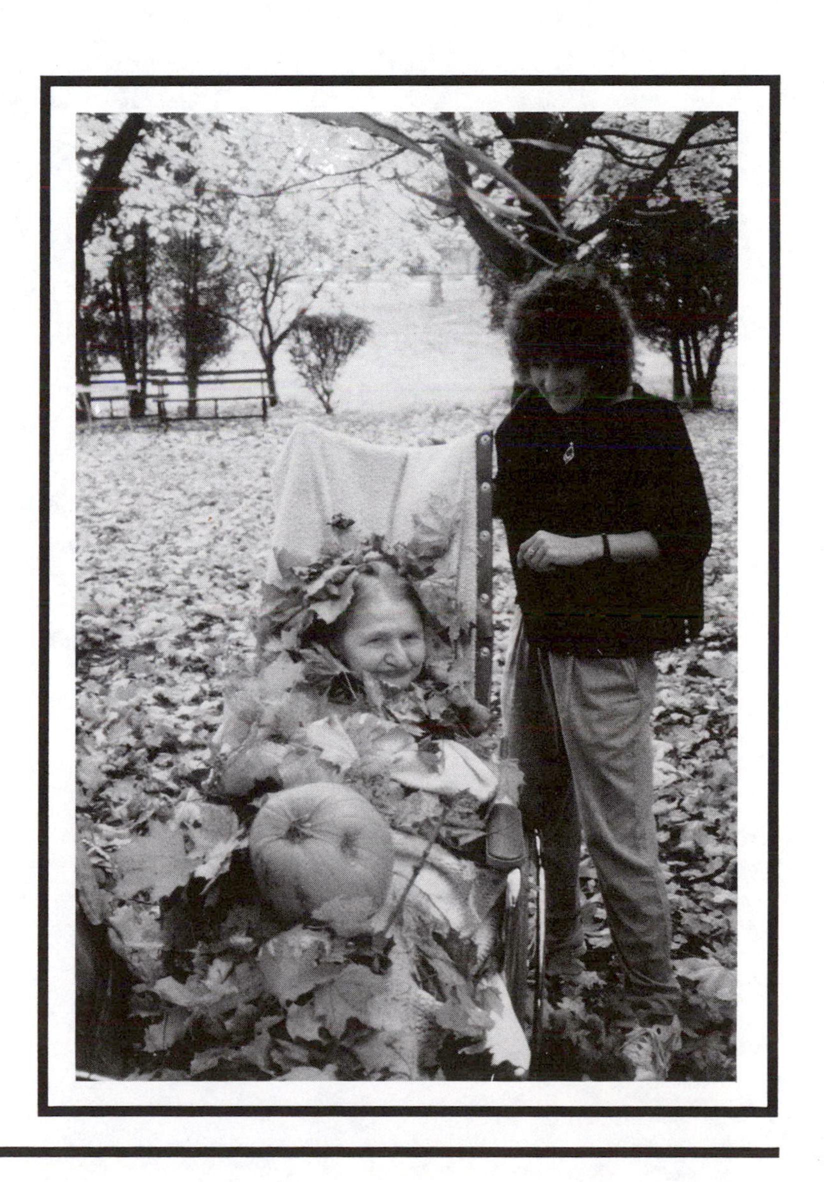

Chapter Two
Therapeutic Recreation and Assessment in the Nursing Home

Assessment is the foundation for all other parts of the therapeutic recreation process. A thorough assessment of each resident is the starting point for developing an individualized needs-based care plan. Every resident has different individual needs. Interventions will be most successful if they are based on these needs. If the therapeutic recreation staff is having difficulty developing a plan of care, or finding activities or interventions that are successful with residents, assessment is the portion of the process that needs more attention.

Assessment is the process of gathering, organizing, and analyzing information in order to gain a full understanding of a resident's past and current levels of functioning, holistic health status, needs, strengths, weaknesses, leisure constraints, and leisure interests for the purpose of making decisions about the treatment plan with the resident, and/or the resident's family. Only after the assessment is completed can areas be identified where change is desirable and possible. The recreation staff's time is at a premium in the nursing home. Frequently the temptation arises to skimp on the assessment process to save time. However, a thorough assessment can be the biggest time saver in the long run. Writing care plans and designing interventions will be much quicker if the staff has a thorough assessment from which to work. An important thing to remember about assessment is that once a system that works for an individual department is developed, stick with it. Some suggestions follow.

What to Assess

There are six areas that should be explored during an assessment. The *first* area is the resident's past and present level of functioning across all domains. The domains of multidimensional assessment usually include areas of physical and mental health, social-emotional functioning, and economic well-being. For therapeutic recreation it is also important to include leisure, occupational, and spiritual areas as well. These authors recommend the following:

1. Physical and Health Status—this includes components such as strength, endurance, flexibility, illness, disability, nutrition, sleep, activities of daily living (e.g., bathing, dressing, grooming, eating, toileting, and mobility), and instrumental activities of daily living (e.g., money management, use of the telephone, travel, shopping, preparing meals, household chores, and medications).
2. Mental Status—this includes the areas of cognitive functioning, attitudes, and motivation as well as any past or present mental health diagnosis such as dementia, Alzheimer's disease, schizophrenia, or psychosis. Also make note if the resident is considered capable of making his or her own decisions.
3. Emotional Status—note present and pervasive feelings: anger, sadness, anxiety, depression or symptoms of depression, happiness, guilt, or shame. Note recent losses including home, possessions, independence, health, friends, or family.

4. Social Status—social resources such as family, friends, organizations, pets, cultural and ethnic ties, and social interaction patterns and skills. Note participation patterns such as active, passive, active (with prompts), or refusal of all interaction. Remember that social interaction is not only one-on-one, but also occurs in small groups or large groups. Avedon (1974) categorizes social interaction patterns by eight categories (see Figure 2.1). Note which of these types of interaction the resident does engage in. Also note social skills such as introducing one's self to other individuals and in a group, comfort level when meeting new people, taking turns, listening, and communication skills. Note the resident's level of comfort when leaving her or his room.
5. Leisure Status—note the resident's level of playfulness, perceptions of competence and control, attitudes toward leisure, level of creativity, level of enjoyment, and depth of involvement in leisure activities. Also note the reasons that the resident engages in leisure activities, such as relaxation, health, excitement, accomplishment/satisfaction, fun/pleasure, relief/escape, companionship, or rejuvenation.
6. Financial Status—note the general financial resources of the resident and any effects this may have on the resident, such as stress or anxiety.
7. Spiritual Status—note any affiliations with religious or spiritual groups and significant beliefs of the resident, such as reincarnation or life after death. Note any concerns the resident mentions such as unresolved spiritual issues, fears of or wishes for death.
8. Occupational Status—note if the resident is retired and how long, past careers, and present feelings of usefulness. Note if the resident would like to continue or begin volunteer work.

The second area that should be assessed is past and present leisure interests. This is usually accomplished by using interest finders (see Figures 2.2 and 2.3, pages 16 and 17, for examples). The resident should be asked to indicate present level of interest as well as past participation level in the activities listed. In the examples shown in Figures 2.2 and 2.3, a 3-point scale is used to indicate level of interest. For the leisure history, a "0" is placed in the box next to activities that the resident never participated in, a "1" denotes participation sometimes, and a "2" indicates frequent participation. Similarly, on the current leisure interest profile, a "0" means no interest, a "1" means some interest, and a "2" means strong interest and a desire to participate frequently. If the resident is unable to complete the interest finder, several options exist. A volunteer, staff member, or family member could assist the resident, or the resident's family could be asked to provide the information if the resident is unable.

When reviewing this information, note significant declines or increases in present interests compared with past interests. Also note the types of activities preferred. For example, a resident may now prefer many outdoor activities, but nothing cultural or social. The therapist should ask himself or herself, "Was the resident interested in cultural and social activities in the past?" Find out why he or she refuses these opportunities now. Comparing past interests and present participation is an important step in the assessment process (see Figure 2.4, page 18).

A third area to be assessed is leisure constraints. Systematically note any constraints that interfere with a resident's leisure participation or interests. For example, a person who has undergone an amputation may not be able to continue her daily nature excursions. Or a person with severe depression may be unable to concentrate, and therefore unable to continue his favorite pastime of reading mysteries. Figure 2.5 (pages 22 and 23) gives an example of a leisure constraints checklist.

Figure 2.1 Social Interaction Patterns

1. Intraindividual—Interaction that takes place within the mind of the individual. Examples: thinking, daydreaming, meditation, prayer, fantasy, imagery, and humming, whistling, singing or talking with oneself.

2. Extraindividual—Interaction that takes place between the individual alone, and her or his environment or objects in the environment. Examples: painting, writing, making a craft, reading, playing solitaire, watching TV, and listening to music when one is alone.

3. Aggregate—Interaction that takes place between the individual and her or his environment in the presence of other people who are also interacting in the same manner. No interaction takes place between the individuals involved. These would be individuals who are engaged in extraindividual interaction all in the same room. Examples: playing bingo, participating in arts and crafts in a group, watching TV or a movie in a group, or listening to music in a group.

4. Interindividual—Competitive or cooperative interaction that takes place between two individuals. Examples: Talking with a friend, talking on the phone, or playing checkers or chess.

5. Unilateral—Interaction between a group and an individual, where the group acts against or listens to the individual. Note if the resident is in the position of the individual or a member of the group. Examples: game of tag, speaking or singing to a group, leading exercise group, leading a discussion or Bible study.

6. Multilateral—Interaction between members of a group, each with the other, with no leader. Examples: poker and other card games, Monopoly, Life, Trivial Pursuit, and other board games.

7. Intragroup—Cooperative interaction between a group of individuals with a common goal. Example: singing in a choir or sing-along and learning new games.

8. Intergroup—Competitive interaction between two groups of individuals. Examples: baseball, basketball, pinochle, bridge, Pictionary, and all team sports.

A fourth area to be assessed is needs. The needs include required physical equipment, issues regarding physical and emotional safety, trust issues, and needs for love and belonging. For example, a resident with dementia may have a physical safety need because of wandering behavior. A person with depression might have emotional safety needs. A person with schizophrenia or dementia may have problems with trust because of paranoia. And a resident without local family or friends may have a need for adopted family to satisfy love and belonging needs.

The final areas to be assessed are the residents' strengths and weaknesses (see Figure 2.6, page 24). For strengths, indicate any strong areas of competence, ability, or interest. For example, a resident may have excellent skills in playing the piano, or crocheting, or have strong interests in photography. These are important to note because they will be assets in the care planning process. Strengths are used as a first choice activity with which to plan interventions. Other strengths include social skills, ability to communicate, ability to make decisions and initiate activity.

For weaknesses, note any strong or pervasive areas of disability or strong dislikes or fears. For example, a diagnosis of dementia would affect the resident's functioning across many domains. Weaknesses are also considered in the care planning process. Sometimes they are the focus of the care plan, while at other times the purpose is to be aware of them and to use the information

Figure 2.2 The Farrington Leisure History

Resident: ______________________ **#:** __________

Room #: ______________________ **Date:** __________

Games

- Billiards
- Bingo
- Baseball/Softball
- Badminton
- Boxing
- Bocce Ball
- Auto Racing
- Checkers
- Croquet
- Chess
- Cards
- Board Games
- Word Finds
- Crossword Puzzles
- Gambling
- Fencing
- Hockey
- Horseshoes
- Quoits
- Jigsaw Puzzles
- Pub Games
- Darts
- Field Hockey
- Football
- Golf
- Horseracing
- Karate/Judo/etc.
- Shuffleboard
- Squash/Handball
- Tennis
- Volleyball
- Archery
- Basketball
- Fitness/Exercise
- Gymnastics
- Table Tennis
- Watching Sports
- Bowling
- Miniature Golf
- Soccer
- Wrestling

Social

- Babysitting
- Club Meetings
- Parties
- Religious Org.
- Shopping
- Social Drinking
- Telephoning
- Volunteering
- Writing Letters
- Ham Radio
- Church
- Encounter Groups
- Night Clubs
- Taverns
- Pets
- Church Suppers
- Dancing
- Dining Out
- Fraternal Orgztn
- Political Activity
- Civic organizations
- Family Parties
- Sitting on Porch
- Visiting Friends
- Volunteer Fire Dept
- Vol. Ambulance
- Auctions

Outdoors

- Driving
- Boating
- Flying
- Gardening
- Jogging
- Motorcycling
- Skindiving
- Diving
- Parachuting
- Surfing
- Go to the Beach
- Water Skiing
- Camping
- Mountain Climbing
- Rollerskating
- Sailing
- Snowmobiling
- ATVs/3-wheelers
- Swimming
- Walking
- Hiking
- Fishing
- Hunting/Trapping
- Bird Watching
- Kite Flying
- Sunbathing
- Bicycling
- Backpacking
- Canoeing
- Riding in a Car
- Horsebackriding
- Iceskating
- Nature Walks
- Parades
- Picnicking
- Rec. Vehicles
- Amusement Parks
- Skiing
- Target Shooting
- Butterfly Watching
- Rock Climbing

Cultural

- Acting
- Carpentry
- Cooking/Baking
- Model Building
- Crafts/Metalwork
- Design Clothes
- Electronics
- Leatherworking
- Needlework
- Plays
- Quilting
- Museums
- Auto Repair
- Antique Cars
- Ceramics
- Collecting
- Crochet
- Decorating
- Draw Houseplans
- Lectures/Educat'n
- Flower Arranging
- Meditation
- Musical Instrument
- Weaving/Knitting
- Creative Writing
- Auto Care
- Bookbinding
- Composing Music
- Poetry
- Repairs/Remodel
- Radio/Music
- Photography
- Sewing
- Concerts
- Traveling
- Antiques
- Movies/TV
- Paint/Draw
- Pottery/Sculpture
- Reading
- Woodworking

Figure 2.3 The Farrington Current Leisure Interest Profile

Resident: ______________________ **#:** __________

Room #: ______________________ **Date:** __________

Games
- [ ] Billiards
- [ ] Bingo
- [ ] Baseball/Softball
- [ ] Badminton
- [ ] Boxing
- [ ] Bocce Ball
- [ ] Auto Racing
- [ ] Checkers
- [ ] Croquet
- [ ] Chess
- [ ] Cards
- [ ] Board Games
- [ ] Word Finds
- [ ] Crossword Puzzles
- [ ] Gambling
- [ ] Fencing
- [ ] Hockey
- [ ] Horseshoes
- [ ] Quoits
- [ ] Jigsaw Puzzles
- [ ] Pub Games
- [ ] Darts
- [ ] Field Hockey
- [ ] Football
- [ ] Golf
- [ ] Horseracing
- [ ] Karate/Judo/etc.
- [ ] Shuffleboard
- [ ] Squash/Handball
- [ ] Tennis
- [ ] Volleyball
- [ ] Archery
- [ ] Basketball
- [ ] Fitness/Exercise
- [ ] Gymnastics
- [ ] Table Tennis
- [ ] Watching Sports
- [ ] Bowling
- [ ] Miniature Golf
- [ ] Soccer
- [ ] Wrestling

Social
- [ ] Babysitting
- [ ] Club Meetings
- [ ] Parties
- [ ] Religious Org.
- [ ] Shopping
- [ ] Social Drinking
- [ ] Telephoning
- [ ] Volunteering
- [ ] Writing Letters
- [ ] Ham Radio
- [ ] Church
- [ ] Encounter Groups
- [ ] Night Clubs
- [ ] Taverns
- [ ] Pets
- [ ] Church Suppers
- [ ] Dancing
- [ ] Dining Out
- [ ] Fraternal Orgztn
- [ ] Political Activity
- [ ] Civic organizations
- [ ] Family Parties
- [ ] Sitting on Porch
- [ ] Visiting Friends
- [ ] Volunteer Fire Dept
- [ ] Vol. Ambulance
- [ ] Auctions

Outdoors
- [ ] Driving
- [ ] Boating
- [ ] Flying
- [ ] Gardening
- [ ] Jogging
- [ ] Motorcycling
- [ ] Skindiving
- [ ] Diving
- [ ] Parachuting
- [ ] Surfing
- [ ] Go to the Beach
- [ ] Water Skiing
- [ ] Camping
- [ ] Mountain Climbing
- [ ] Rollerskating
- [ ] Sailing
- [ ] Snowmobiling
- [ ] ATVs/3-wheelers
- [ ] Swimming
- [ ] Walking
- [ ] Hiking
- [ ] Fishing
- [ ] Hunting/Trapping
- [ ] Bird Watching
- [ ] Kite Flying
- [ ] Sunbathing
- [ ] Bicycling
- [ ] Backpacking
- [ ] Canoeing
- [ ] Riding in a Car
- [ ] Horsebackriding
- [ ] Iceskating
- [ ] Nature Walks
- [ ] Parades
- [ ] Picnicking
- [ ] Rec. Vehicles
- [ ] Amusement Parks
- [ ] Skiing
- [ ] Target Shooting
- [ ] Butterfly Watching
- [ ] Rock Climbing

Cultural
- [ ] Acting
- [ ] Carpentry
- [ ] Cooking/Baking
- [ ] Model Building
- [ ] Crafts/Metalwork
- [ ] Design Clothes
- [ ] Electronics
- [ ] Leatherworking
- [ ] Needlework
- [ ] Plays
- [ ] Quilting
- [ ] Museums
- [ ] Auto Repair
- [ ] Antique Cars
- [ ] Ceramics
- [ ] Collecting
- [ ] Crochet
- [ ] Decorating
- [ ] Draw Houseplans
- [ ] Lectures/Educat'n
- [ ] Flower Arranging
- [ ] Meditation
- [ ] Musical Instrument
- [ ] Weaving/Knitting
- [ ] Creative Writing
- [ ] Auto Care
- [ ] Bookbinding
- [ ] Composing Music
- [ ] Poetry
- [ ] Repairs/Remodel
- [ ] Radio/Music
- [ ] Photography
- [ ] Sewing
- [ ] Concerts
- [ ] Traveling
- [ ] Antiques
- [ ] Movies/TV
- [ ] Paint/Draw
- [ ] Pottery/Sculpture
- [ ] Reading
- [ ] Woodworking

Figure 2.4 Leisure Interests and Needs

Resident Name ______________________________

Resident #: ______________

Room #: ____________ Birth Date: ______________ Date: _________

Part I. Leisure Interest Types

Directions: Rate the following types of leisure activities in order of your preference on a scale of 1 to 10.

#1 = Most Preferred #10 = Least Preferred

☐ Arts and Crafts
☐ Educational
☐ Games
☐ Outdoors and Nature
☐ Sports and Exercise
☐ Collecting
☐ Cultural, including Art and Music
☐ Socializing and Visiting
☐ Clubs and Organizations
☐ Volunteering

Part II. Leisure Needs

Directions: Rate the following reasons as to their importance in your selection of leisure activities on a scale of 1 to 8.

#1 = Most Important #8 = Least Important

☐ Relaxation
☐ Excitement
☐ Fun
☐ Companionship
☐ Health
☐ Accomplishment
☐ Escape
☐ Rejuvenation

Resident/Family Signature: ______________________ Date: __________

TR Signature: __________________________ Date: __________

accordingly in planning an intervention. For instance, if a resident has a strong fear of animals, proper care planning would avoid placement of the resident in a pet therapy program. Another example would be a resident who lost a child and has unresolved grief *may* not be suited for a program with children. All of the information gathered during the assessment will be pulled together into a plan of care for the individual resident. In this way, the plan of care will be need-based and individualized. These are two important requirements for successful care plans. See Figure 2.7 (pages 25 and 26) for an example of a report format for the assessment.

How To Do An Assessment: Sources of Information

The information needed for a thorough assessment can be gathered from several sources. The more sources used, the more complete and accurate the information will be. Most of the information will come from the resident if she or he is able to communicate. The assessment process is a partnership with the resident and should be completed with the resident when possible. If the resident is unable to communicate, visiting family and friends may be valuable sources of information. Families and friends can also help the TR staff gather information from the resident. For example, a family member can assist the resident in completing the past and present interest inventories. This will save time for the TR staff while providing an opportunity for the family and the resident to learn more about each other. Information can also be gathered from other health professionals such as nursing staff, physical therapy, the physician, dietary staff, and social services staff. Finally, much of the information needed can be gathered from the resident's medical record or chart.

There are several ways to gather the information. The most popular method is interviewing. This is simply asking questions and then listening carefully to the answers. Information should also be gathered by observing the resident in activities and in social interactions with family, friends, and other residents. Tests are sometimes used to gather information. For example, the Mini Mental State test and the geriatric depression scale are frequently administered in the nursing home. Information can be taken from these tests for the assessment. Finally, information can be gathered by using checklists and questionnaires, such as interest finders. It is important to note in your documentation where the information came from and how it was gathered.

Documentation of Assessment

The results of your assessment should be summarized and placed on the resident's medical chart in the therapeutic recreation section. Figure 2.7 gives an example of an assessment summary. Actual interest finders, constraints assessments, and other tools used in gathering information may be placed in the medical record for future reference. There should be a section under therapeutic recreation clearly marked "ASSESSMENT." There should be another section under TR marked "RESIDENT DATA" where it is wise to include a resident data sheet with general information that is needed by the TR staff, e.g., does the resident smoke, drink, have sensitivity to sun, or have any food allergies or salient medical conditions such as diabetes. Copies of this form are found in Figure 2.7. Also, the activity section of the MDS (Minimum Data Set, see page 71) must be

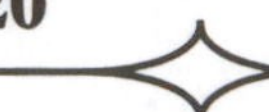

completed with input from the TR staff. The results of the assessment should always be discussed with the resident, when possible, or with the family. Always document when this has occurred in the "PROGRESS NOTES" and what input the resident or family had regarding the results of the assessment. Use their actual comments when possible. An entry in the progress notes should also be made noting the date the assessment was completed, and the next scheduled assessment or review. It should refer the reader to the results and give the location of the actual summary in the chart while providing a concise summary of the results and plan of action. Always review the resident's medications and current diagnoses and note this in the progress note. Also review activity participation records (flow sheets) and note the general trends in the progress note on assessment.

Other Measures

Several other tests have been found helpful in assessment process for nursing home residents. The Multidimensional Observation Scale for Elderly Subjects (MOSES) is reported as a reliable and valid means of assessing cognitive and psychosocial functioning of older adults (Helmes, Csapo, & Short, 1987). It is a 40-item test that assesses five areas of functioning: self-care functioning, disoriented behavior, depressed/anxious mood, irritable behavior, and withdrawn behavior. All of these areas are important in the provision of recreation therapy.

The Timed Manual Performance Instrument is another more direct indicator of overall function. A section of the test that was utilized in recent nursing home research is known as the "Doors Test" (Buettner, 1994). Each resident is evaluated closing a variety of fasteners that are commonly found in the home. These fasteners are mounted on nine hinged doors (in a 3 x 3 array) on a 2 x 3 foot plywood panel that attaches to a table. Residents sit in front of the panel and are timed as they attempt to close each fastener. The fasteners are closed in numerical sequence, using the following format, which is read to the resident. "This is door number ___. It is closed like this (demonstrate). Do you have any questions about how to close door number ___? Place your hands on the table please. When I say 'go' close door number ___ and latch it up tight. Ready? GO." The timing begins from the last word "go" and ends when the door is completely latched. Add the total time for all nine doors (see Figure 2.8, page 27).

The Mini Mental State test is the most widely used cognitive assessment in both research and cognitive settings. It was developed by Folstein and colleagues (1975) and is a good indicator of cognitive impairment. The test is scored on a 30-point scale, with a score of less than 17 indicating significant cognitive impairment.

The modified-for-wheelchair Wells Sit-and-Reach test (Flexibility Test) has been used successfully to monitor progress for exercise and sensorimotor therapy programs (Buettner, 1989 and 1994). On this test the resident sits with her feet against the vertical support, knees as straight as possible, and reaches forward with both arms sliding a movable bar with her fingertips (see Figure 2.9, page 27). The residents should have the opportunity to "warm up" for 5 to 10 minutes before taking this test. For uniformity the following statement should be read to the resident: "This is a test to find out how far you can reach. You should keep your knees straight and slide the bar as far as you can. I will show you how it works." Give a demonstration.

Another useful indicator for exercise or sensorimotor interventions is the grip strength test (see Figure 2.10, page 28). A bulb-type hand dynamometer should be used since older adults often have an arthritic grip. Each resident in the program is tested first for strength in the right grip, and then in the left grip. The bulb of the dynamometer is placed between the palm of the hand and the first and second joints of the fingers. The dial should be facing the therapist. During the test the hands should not be allowed to touch any other object. A squeezing movement down with the elbow slightly bent is demonstrated first by the therapist. The dial should be read to the nearest pound of pressure on the gauge. The following cues should be read to each resident taking the grip strength test: "This ball must fit into your hand like this (demonstrate). On the count of three you should squeeze as hard as you can. One-two-three SQUEEZE!" Repeat the test with the other hand.

The Geriatric Depression Scale is a quick and easy self-reported 15-item questionnaire. Questions examine issues such as:

- Have you dropped many of your activities or interests?
- Do you often get bored?
- Do you prefer to stay in your room rather than going out?

A score of 5 or more indicates depression may be present. This tool has demonstrated sensitivity for detecting major depression in older adults. It is not a valid tool for residents with cognitive impairments (Birren, Sloane, & Cohen, 1992).

Figure 2.5 Comprehensive Leisure Constraints Assessment

SCORING KEY: 0 = NO X = YES

Resident: ______________________ **Assessment Date:** ______________

Physical Constraints:

- [ ] Impaired mobility
- [ ] Uses wheelchair
- [ ] Uses cane or walker
- [ ] Uses gerichair
- [ ] Amputation
- [ ] Prosthesis
- [ ] Needs assistance w/ mobility
- [ ] Unsteady gait
- [ ] Needs assistance w/ transfer
- [ ] Non-weightbearing
- [ ] Paralysis: ____________
- [ ] Usually not out of bed
- [ ] Contractures
- [ ] Independently mobile
- [ ] Ambulates: ____________
- [ ] Difficulty eating: ____________
- [ ] Needs assistance with eating
- [ ] Feeding tube
- [ ] Need to lose weight
- [ ] Nausea
- [ ] Vertigo or dizziness
- [ ] Sleeps during day
- [ ] Frequent naps
- [ ] Awake at night
- [ ] Impaired range of motion
- [ ] Impaired fine motor skills
- [ ] Impaired gross motor skills
- [ ] Reduced endurance
- [ ] Tires easily
- [ ] Complains of pain
- [ ] Incontinence
- [ ] Catheter or Colostomy
- [ ] Uses oxygen
- [ ] Dialysis
- [ ] Needs assistance w/ ADLs
- [ ] Other: ____________

Environmental/Situational Constraints:

- [ ] Limited financial resources
- [ ] Decline in health status
- [ ] Ecological barriers
- [ ] Lacks equipment for activity
- [ ] Needs to adjust to placement
- [ ] Lacks leisure skills
- [ ] Unaware of leisure activities
- [ ] Unable to adapt leisure
- [ ] Limited time for leisure
- [ ] Architectural barriers
- [ ] Disturbed by noise
- [ ] Other: ____________

Sensory Constraints:

- [ ] Vision impairment
- [ ] Smell impairment
- [ ] Taste impairment
- [ ] Tactile impairment
- [ ] Hearing impairment
- [ ] Other: ____________

Communication Constraints:

- [ ] Difficulty speaking
- [ ] Unable to read or write
- [ ] Difficulty being understood
- [ ] Unable to communicate
- [ ] Refuses to communicate
- [ ] Difficulty hearing
- [ ] Uses a hearing aid
- [ ] Alternative communication
- [ ] Foreign language primary
- [ ] English primary
- [ ] Converses with others
- [ ] Receptive to conversation
- [ ] Initiates conversation
- [ ] Initiates topics
- [ ] Other: ____________

Interpersonal Constraints:

- [ ] Difficulty imagining
- [ ] Difficulty interacting w/ object
- [ ] Difficulty w/ aggregation
- [ ] Difficulty w/ 1 : 1 interaction
- [ ] Difficulty w/ unilateral
- [ ] Difficulty w/ multilateral
- [ ] Difficulty w/ cooperation
- [ ] Difficulty making eye contact
- [ ] Few facial expressions
- [ ] Withdrawn
- [ ] Refuses social interaction
- [ ] Anxiety in group settings
- [ ] Dislikes social interaction
- [ ] Prefers to interact w/ staff
- [ ] Difficult interaction w/ residents
- [ ] Refuses contact w/ residents
- [ ] Unassertive
- [ ] Difficulty initiating interaction
- [ ] Passive participation
- [ ] Active participation
- [ ] Difficulty waiting turn
- [ ] Difficulty making new friends
- [ ] Poor appearance
- [ ] Lacks friends
- [ ] Has many friends
- [ ] Manipulative
- [ ] Enjoys pets

Additional Comments:

TR Signature: ______________________ **Date:** ______________

Figure 2.5 Comprehensive Leisure Constraints Assessment (continued)

Emotional and Attitude Constraints:

- Flat effect/no expression
- Unable to identify feelings
- Unable to express feelings
- Blanket emotional response
- Unable to identify own needs
- Prior psychiatric diagnosis
- History of abuse
- History of addiction
- Present psychiatric diagnosis
- Taking psychotropic meds
- Does not enjoy activities
- Lacks motivation
- Prefers to do nothing
- Reduced activity level
- Refuses activity participation
- Resists new experiences
- Refuses to plan on leisure
- Does not value leisure
- Does not enjoy leisure
- Low self esteem
- Lacks own identity
- Dependent on others
- Lacks confidence in abilities
- Feelings of worthlessness
- Dissatisfied with own life
- Lacks spirituality or religion
- Questions meaning of life
- Anxiety about leaving room
- Anxious/nervous/panic
- Feelings of fear
- Feelings of paranoia
- Hallucinations
- Difficulty identifying choices
- Feels little choice
- Difficulty making choices
- External locus of control
- Feelings of helplessness
- External source of evaluation
- Feelings of guilt
- Multiple losses/recent grief
- Feels sad
- Cries
- Feels tired much of the time
- Frequently irritable
- Feels angry
- Outbursts of rage
- Lack of pleasure
- Lack of interest (apathetic)
- Feels discontented frequently
- Frequent complaints
- Negative outlook
- Difficulty being playful
- Lacks feelings of competence
- Lacks feelings of control
- Dissatisfied w/ own leisure
- Unrealistic self expectations
- Other: ________________

Cognitive Status:

- Unresponsive to stimulus
- Unable to identify objects
- Unable to identify colors
- Unable to identify shapes
- Unable to categorize objects
- Unable to recall recent events
- Unable to recall past events
- Unable to solve math probs
- Unable to follow directions
- Unable to pair objects
- Unable to pair words
- Memory problems
- Responds appropriately
- Repetitive speech
- Repetitive motion
- Rambling/incoherent speech
- Uses nonsense words
- Smiles inappropriately
- Laughs inappropriately
- Short attention span
- Confused
- Unable to focus attention
- Difficulty understanding
- Not oriented x 3
- Enjoys reminiscing about past
- Unable to copy patterns
- Unable to state own name
- Not responsive to own name
- Unable to identify family
- Unable to identify TR staff
- Unable to locate own room
- Unable to locate activities
- Recent change in medication
- Recent change in room, etc.
- Recent hospitalization
- Recent infection
- Recent fall/head injury
- Sudden change in cognition
- Other: ________________

Family Interaction:

- Does not have family
- Family at a distance
- Little or no family contact
- Res. desires more autonomy
- Family is controlling
- Family is argumentative
- Family has frequent complaints
- Difficult family interaction
- Has few family members
- Recent family loss/grief (2yr)
- Family does not share leisure
- Other: ________________

Behavior Problems:

- Involuntary movements
- Inappropriate body exposure
- Physically abusive to self
- Physically combative
- Trespasses
- Repeated questions/phrases
- Noisy/Disruptive
- Demanding staff
- Argumentative
- Aggressive
- Easily agitated
- Impatient
- Easily frustrated
- Refuses care or meds
- Refuses to respond
- Verbally abusive
- Paces/Restless
- Wanders/Elopes
- Dangerous to self or others
- Takes others' things
- Other: ________________

TR Signature: ______________________________ **Date:** ________________

Figure 2.6 The Farrington Strengths Assessment

SCORING KEY: 0 = NO; X = YES

Resident: ____________________ **Assessment Date:** ____________

PHYSICAL STRENGTHS:

- ☐ Independently mobile
- ☐ Ambulates ad lib
- ☐ Enjoys eating
- ☐ Independent ADLs
- ☐ Endurance
- ☐ Strength
- ☐ Flexibility
- ☐ Range of motion
- ☐ Fine motor skills
- ☐ Gross motor skills
- ☐ Other: ____________

ENVIRONMENTAL/SITUATIONAL STRENGTHS:

- ☐ Financial resources
- ☐ Health status
- ☐ Enjoys leisure activities
- ☐ Adjusting to placement
- ☐ Values leisure
- ☐ Awareness of leisure activities
- ☐ Adequate time for leisure
- ☐ Able to adapt to leisure
- ☐ Other: ____________

SENSORY STRENGTHS:

- ☐ Vision
- ☐ Smell
- ☐ Taste
- ☐ Touch
- ☐ Hearing
- ☐ Other: ____________

COMMUNICATIONS STRENGTHS:

- ☐ Speech
- ☐ Reading
- ☐ Writing
- ☐ Uses a hearing aid
- ☐ Alternative communication
- ☐ English primary
- ☐ Enjoys conversation
- ☐ Initiates conversation
- ☐ Initiates topics

INTERPERSONAL STRENGTHS:

- ☐ Imagination
- ☐ Interaction w/ object
- ☐ Aggregate
- ☐ 1:1 interaction
- ☐ Unilateral
- ☐ Multilateral
- ☐ Cooperation
- ☐ Competition
- ☐ Makes eye contact
- ☐ Uses facial expressions
- ☐ Enjoys social interaction
- ☐ Enjoys small group settings
- ☐ Enjoys large group settings
- ☐ Likes to interact w/ staff
- ☐ Interacts w/ residents
- ☐ Gets along with roommate
- ☐ Assertive
- ☐ Initiates interaction
- ☐ Passive participation
- ☐ Active participation
- ☐ Makes new friends
- ☐ Appearance
- ☐ Family and/or friends
- ☐ Enjoys pets

EMOTIONAL & ATTITUDE STRENGTHS:

- ☐ Able to identify feelings
- ☐ Expressive feelings
- ☐ Able to identify own needs
- ☐ Has motivation
- ☐ Prefers to be active
- ☐ Enjoys new experiences
- ☐ Plans own leisure
- ☐ Internal source of evaluation
- ☐ Positive self-esteem
- ☐ Strong identity
- ☐ Independent
- ☐ Satisfied with own life
- ☐ Spirituality or religion
- ☐ Able to identify choices
- ☐ Able to make choices
- ☐ Internal locus of control
- ☐ Playfulness
- ☐ Enjoys pleasure
- ☐ Shows interest/curiosity
- ☐ Creative
- ☐ Positive attitude
- ☐ Feels competence
- ☐ Feels control
- ☐ Enjoys humor

COGNITIVE STRENGTHS:

- ☐ Enjoys reminiscing
- ☐ Able to identify objects
- ☐ Able to identify colors
- ☐ Able to identify shapes
- ☐ Able to categorize objects
- ☐ Able to recall past events
- ☐ Able to solve math problems
- ☐ Able to follow directions
- ☐ Able to pair objects
- ☐ Able to pair words
- ☐ Knows own name
- ☐ Oriented x 3
- ☐ Able to identify family
- ☐ Able to identify staff
- ☐ Able to locate own room

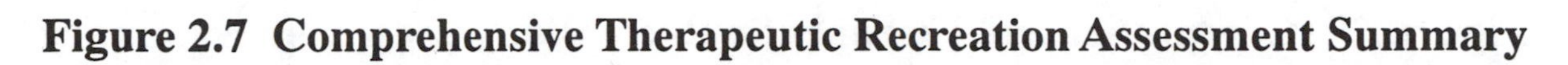

Figure 2.7 Comprehensive Therapeutic Recreation Assessment Summary

Resident: ______________________ **#:** __________

Room #: __________ **Date:** ______________

Summary of Functioning Levels

Physical: ______________________

Mental: ______________________

Emotional: ______________________

Social: ______________________

Financial: ______________________

Spiritual: ______________________

Occupational: ______________________

LEISURE

Control: ______________________

Competence: ______________________

Attitudes: ______________________

Playfulness: ______________________

Participation: ______________________

Needs:

- ☐ Relaxation
- ☐ Companionship
- ☐ Escape
- ☐ Health
- ☐ Accomplishment
- ☐ Rejuvenation
- ☐ Excitement
- ☐ Fun

Leisure Interests

Major Past Interests: ______________________

Major Current Interests: ______________________

Comparision of Past and Present and Types: ______________________

Figure 2.7 Comprehensive Therapeutic Recreation Assessment Summary (continued)

Leisure Constraints

Intraindividual Constraints

Physical: ______

Environmental: ______

Sensory: ______

Extraindividual Constraints

Communication: ______

Interpersonal: ______

Family: ______

Behavioral: ______

Interindividual Constraints

Emotional: ______

Attitudes: ______

Cognative: ______

Needs

Physical: ______

Safety and Trust: ______

Love and Belonging: ______

Strengths	Weaknesses

TR Signature: ______ Date: ______

Resident/Family Signature: ______ Date: ______

Figure 2.8 Timed Manual Performance Test

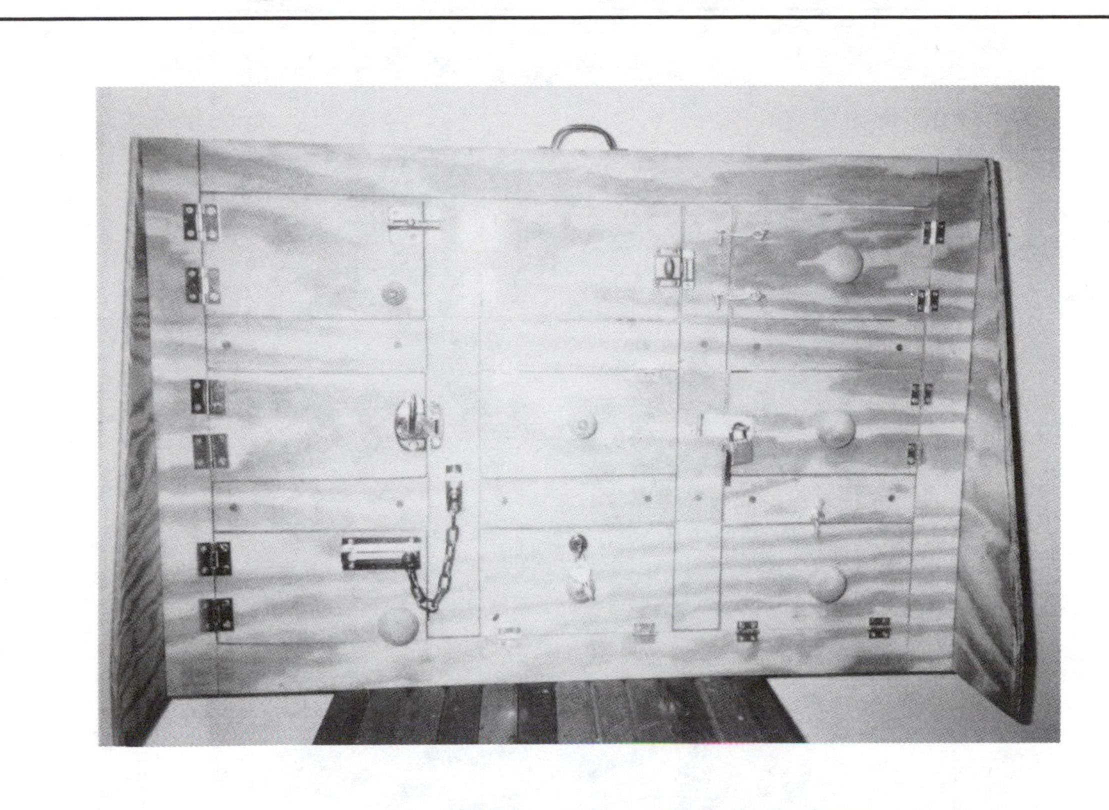

Figure 2.9 Flexibility Test

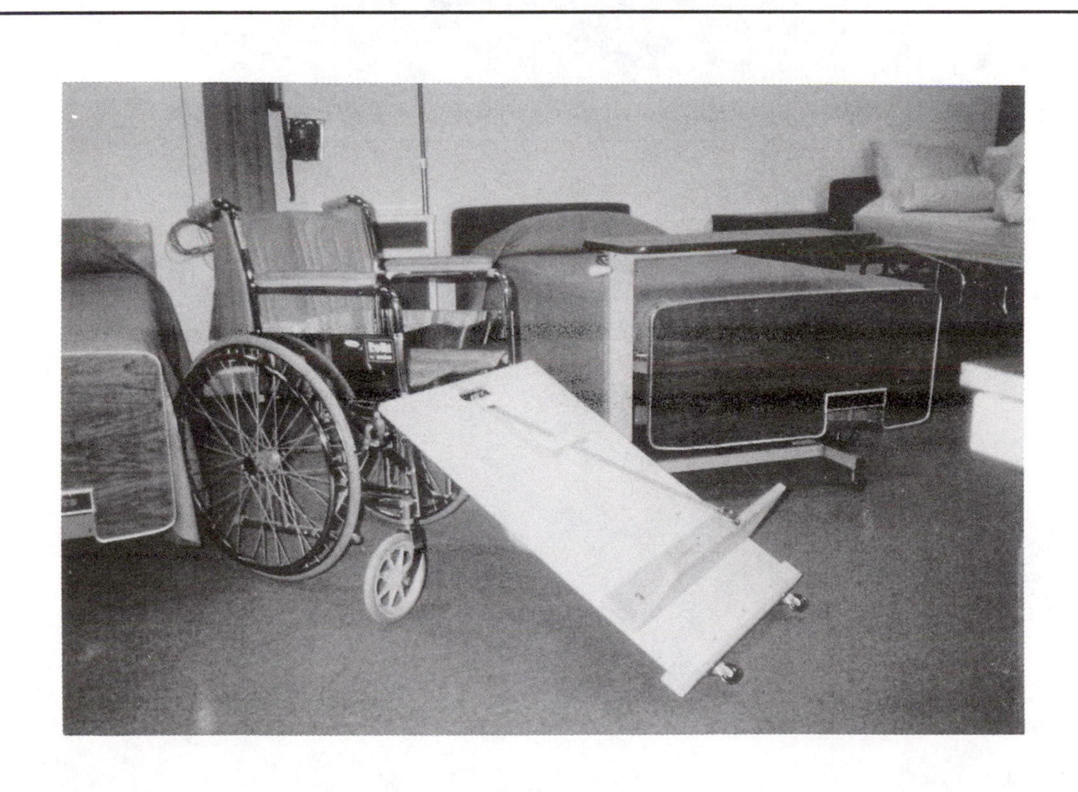

Figure 2.10 Grip Strength Test

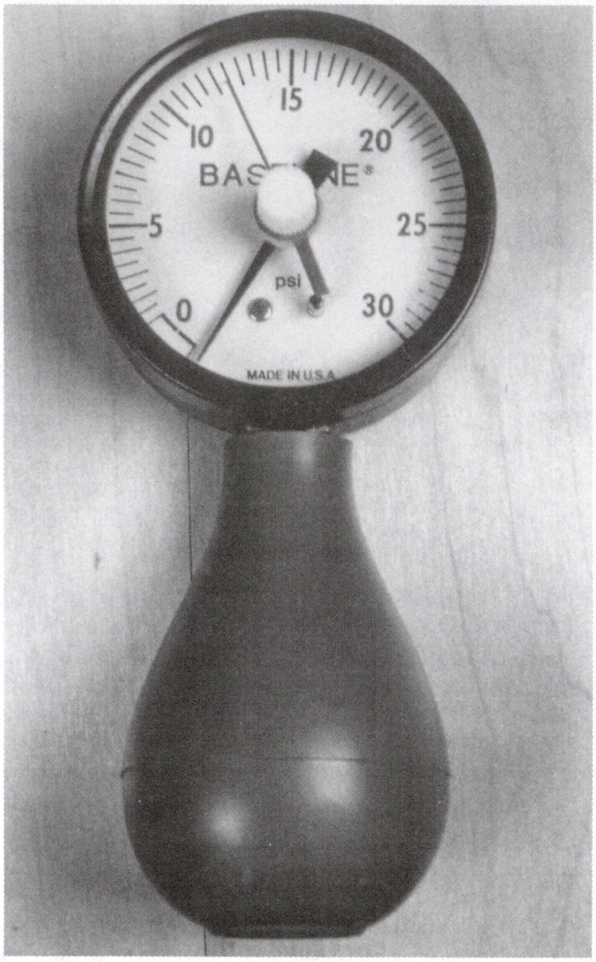

Section Two

Planning

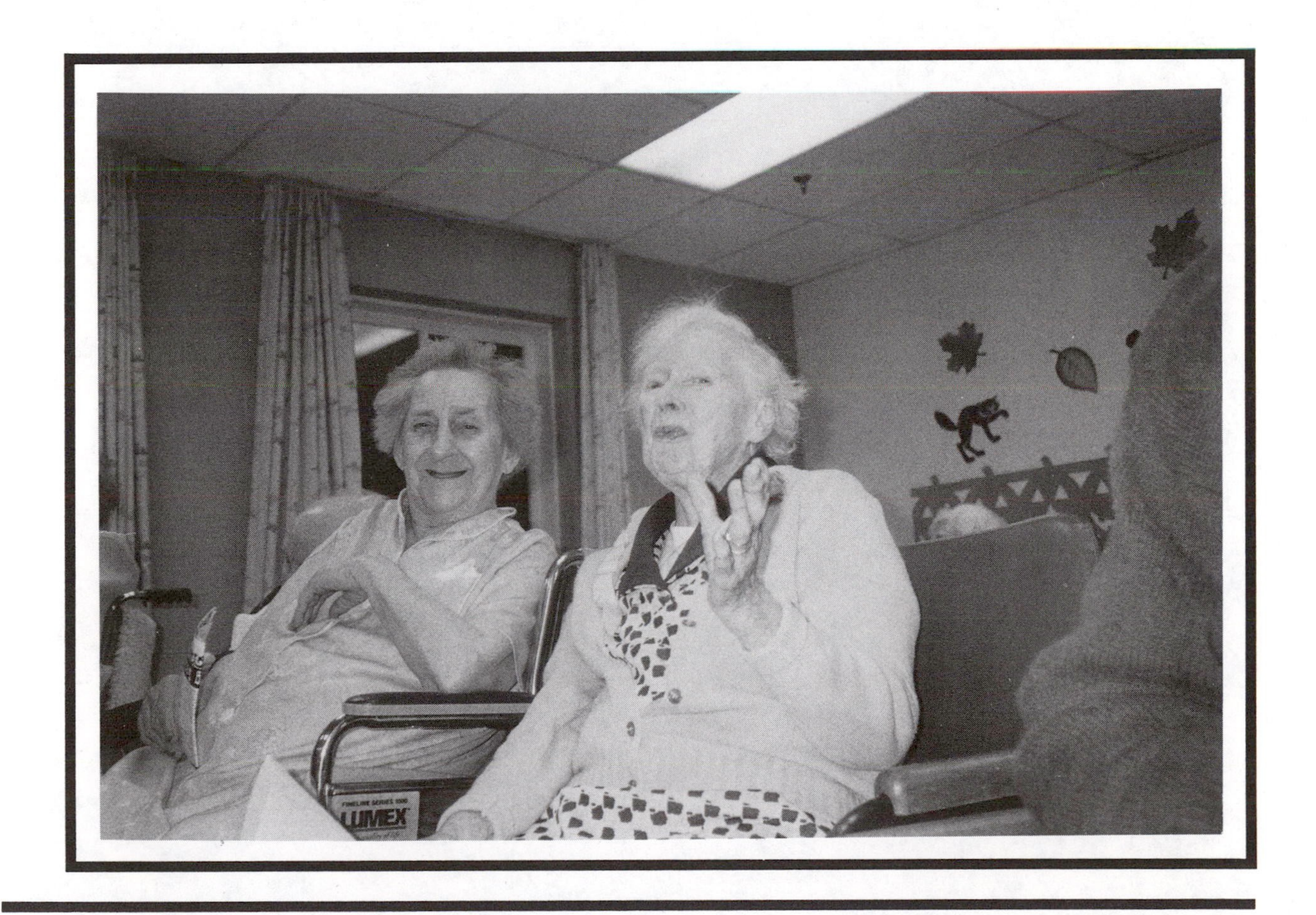

Chapter Three

Goal Planning

The information gathered in the assessment process is the basis of the care plan. The next step in the process is to organize the assessment material so that it can be helpful in goal planning. From the results of your assessment, including the MDS, list all of the resident's problems and needs. Next list the resident's strengths, including current leisure interests that are strong. Then, evaluate each problem/need according to the following criteria. Eliminate problems and needs that do not meet the criteria by crossing them off the list. Flag problems/needs that meet as many of the criteria as possible. These will be the problems/needs that will be considered for intervention. This process will be most accurate if it is actually written out on paper as opposed to "thinking it through" in one's mind.

Evaluation criteria:

1. Will progress made on this problem/need significantly improve the resident's quality of life? (What are the benefits?)
2. Can this problem/need be addressed in a therapeutic recreation/leisure activity?
3. Is there a strength that the resident has that could be used in the intervention to increase chances of success?
4. What is the likelihood of a positive outcome from intervention with this particular problem/need? (Is change possible or likely?)
5. Does the resident think it is a problem?
6. Is the resident willing to make changes in this area?
7. What does the resident want to work on?

Generally, the therapeutic recreation staff should select no more than three goals per resident at one time. Working on more than three goals at one time is extremely difficult, time consuming, and confusing to both the resident and staff. Any problems that have been triggered on the MDS should receive priority consideration when completing this evaluation. The purpose of this process is to select the problem/need that will most benefit the resident's quality of life and respond best to a therapeutic recreation intervention. Successful outcomes are more likely when problems/needs are paired with a strength during the intervention. The goal of this evaluation process is to narrow down the list of problems/needs to no more than three. It is important that the resident has input in this phase of the process. Her wishes should be considered above all others. Choosing a goal that the resident is interested in will maximize successful outcomes. Input from other staff and departments is essential as well, particularly if the intervention will involve that department.

Note that the problem/need does not have to be directly related to leisure or activity, though it may be. The problem/need may be physical, emotional, behavioral, spiritual, or from any other domain. Remember that therapeutic recreation is used to improve health and wellness using interventions in recreational or leisure activities. It is the intervention that is related to leisure, not necessarily the problem. Chapter Four is an example of this part of the planning process using a case study of a nursing home resident.

Writing Goals and Objectives

After choosing the problems and needs to be addressed and then choosing the strengths that will be used to address them, the next step is to write the goals, objectives, and performance measures. The goal is stated in terms of what the resident will be able to do when he or she successfully completes the intervention. This is the general behavioral outcome of the intervention program. For example, the resident will demonstrate the ability to engage in an extraindividual activity (engage in an interaction with an object by herself). The therapist must consider what the resident will be able to do if the intervention is successful and state it clearly and simply. This is the goal.

Objectives are specific behaviors that the resident will learn or do to reach the general goal. There are usually at least 3—no more than 10—objectives for each goal. The question, what are the steps necessary for the resident (or staff) to accomplish this goal, must be answered. To be concise about who is responsible for each objective is imperative. For example, for the above goal, some objectives would be:

1. The staff will use leisure education to teach the concept of extraindividual activities to the resident.
2. The resident will be able to identify extraindividual activities.
3. The resident will create a list of extraindividual activities that she would be willing to try.
4. The resident will choose at least three of the activities to try within the next 90 days.
5. The staff will provide the necessary materials in the resident's room for the activities selected.
6. The resident will choose specific times within 90 days to try each activity at least three times by herself in her room (nine sessions).
7. The therapeutic recreation staff will ask the resident to evaluate her experience after each activity, using a scale of 1 (low) to 5 (high), to measure the following dimensions: depth of involvement, enjoyment, competence, and control. The staff will also keep a record of the duration of these activities.

Finally, a performance measure is established for each goal. This measure will specify the exact criteria to determine if the goal has been achieved. The performance measure should contain a date by which the goal is to be met and reevaluated. It should specify who will decide if the goal has been met, and what the exact standards are for judging the behavior. This part of the goal answers the question, "How and when will we know if the goal has been met?" For example, completion of the nine evaluations of the activity sessions mentioned above will be taken as evidence that the goal has been completed. The goal will be reevaluated in 90 days by the TR staff and the resident.

The goal, objectives, and performance measure are generally documented in the interdisciplinary care plan. It is good practice to refer to the general goal in the progress note and to refer the reader to the care plan (see Figure 3.1) for the objectives and performance measure. The progress note should contain a short justification as to why the goal was selected, and should refer to the assessment in which the problem or need was identified.

Figure 3.1 The Farrington Therapeutic Recreation Plan of Care

Resident: ______________________ **#:** __________

Room #: __________ **DOB:** __________ **Date:** __________

Problem/Needs List	Strengths List
1.	1.
2.	2.
3.	3.
4.	4.
5.	5.

Care Plan

Goal	Performance Measure	Objectives/Intervention

Therapeutic Interventions Recommended:

- [ ] Newcomer Group
- [ ] Remotivation
- [ ] Sensory Stimulation
- [ ] Guided Imagery
- [ ] Horticulture Therapy
- [ ] Art Therapy
- [ ] Leisure Education
- [ ] Reminiscing
- [ ] Assertiveness Training
- [ ] Hug Therapy
- [ ] Grief Group
- [ ] Reality Orientation
- [ ] Relaxation
- [ ] Pet Therapy
- [ ] Music Therapy
- [ ] Validation
- [ ] Values Clarification
- [ ] Empowerment
- [ ] Resocialization
- [ ] Humor

Signature: ______________________ Date: __________

EXAMPLE: Mr. B. just entered the nursing home. He did not identify any leisure skills or interests during his assessment interview. His goal is: Mr. B. will improve his leisure skills. He did, however, voice an interest in learning to play some of the games in the lounge. Building on this interest, the objectives for Mr. B. may be:

(1) Mr. B. will meet with his therapist to discuss specific leisure interests and options 15 minutes daily over the next 3 days.
(2) Mr. B. will choose one game or activity from the leisure interest board to learn.
(3) Mr. B. will demonstrate the ability to play the game or take part in the activity within the next 30 days.

The sequence of objectives exemplifies goal attainment scaling. To test the measurability of an objective, put the objective in question form:

Did Mr. B. meet with the therapist to discuss specific "interests?" "Yes" or "no."

Figure 3.2 Verbs to Use When Writing Objectives

Action verbs are usually used when writing objectives. Some useful verbs include:

Knowledge	Comprehension	Application	Synthesis	Analysis
arrange	classify	apply	arrange	categorize
define	describe	choose	assemble	compare
duplicate	discuss	demonstrate	construct	inspect
label	explain	illustrate	collect	contrast
match	identify	shop	plan	solve
list	indicate	sketch	prepare	examine
name	locate	interpret	create	question
order	select	schedule	propose	test
recognize	translate	practice	manage	distinguish
repeat	restate	employ	design	criticize
recall	express	operate	write	inventory

In summary, goals and objectives are statements that give direction to recreation therapy treatment. They must be realistic and achievable to enable the therapist and the resident to experience success. The process of revising and updating goals and objectives is inherent to the care planning process.

SAMPLE GOALS AND OBJECTIVES

Condition or Problem:
Resident will not communicate.

Goal:
Resident will verbally make needs and desires known.

Objectives:
1. Resident will respond directly to short questions with prompting.
2. Resident will respond directly to short questions without prompting.
3. Resident will engage in a 5-minute conversation one time daily with prompting.
4. Resident will initiate a 5-minute conversation during each social program.

Condition or Problem:
Resident is unable to manage his anger.

Goal:
Resident will identify his feelings of anger when they occur.

Objectives:
1. Resident will report each week to the therapist each time he felt another resident picked on or bothered him.
2. Resident will keep a list of things he thinks he should not feel and report these feelings to the therapist.
3. Resident will identify instances when he felt picked on about something and discuss how that felt.
4. Resident will identify situations that make him angry.

Condition or Problem:
Resident has poor self-acceptance/self-esteem. The resident makes no eye contact with others in the unit.

Goal:
Resident will demonstrate eye contact while communicating with others.

Objectives:
1. The resident will talk about looking at others with her primary therapist.
2. Resident will demonstrate eye contact while discussing topics that are not personal.
3. Resident will demonstrate eye contact with one other person during a social program.

Condition or Problem:
The resident does not solve problems or make simple decisions.

Goal:
Resident will make decisions about her daily activities.

Objectives:
1. Resident will list two or three activities that are available to her while looking at the activity schedule.
2. Resident will choose one activity that she would like to participate in.
3. Resident will participate in the activity.
4. Resident will report to the recreation therapist how she felt about her decision.
5. Resident will make a decision regarding attending the program again based on her feelings.

Condition or Problem:
Poor social functioning. Resident is withdrawn, spending most of her time alone in her room, watching television. She has no close friends and does not trust staff.

Goal:

Resident will socially interact with others.

Objectives:

1. Resident will take a walk daily for at least 10 minutes.
2. Resident will speak to one person while on her walk.
3. Resident will telephone her recreation therapist for 5 minutes between 11:30 a.m. and noon.
4. Resident will identify leisure interests with her therapist.
5. Resident will tell her therapist of her plan to attend one leisure time activity during the week.
6. Resident will attend a social program one time per week.

Condition or Problem:

Social isolation. Because of disorientation and confusion, the resident has isolated himself.

Goal:

Resident will participate in a small group program.

Objectives:

1. Resident will demonstrate improved concentration as evidenced by sustained attention on task for 10 minutes per session.
2. Resident will demonstrate the ability to follow a 2-step instruction during each activity.
3. Resident will initiate a 5-minute conversation at the end of the activity session to talk about the project.

Condition or Problem:

Lack of motivation to participate.

Goal:

Resident will participate in leisure activities.

Objectives:

1. Resident will have self-directed leisure behavior as demonstrated by engaging in an activity in the leisure lounge.
2. Resident will attend one program daily for 2 weeks as jointly determined by the resident and the treatment team.
3. The resident will choose and attend one additional activity for a month.
4. Resident will look through the paper and select several community activities he would like to attend.
5. Resident and therapist will attend one community function weekly from those listed in the paper for 1 month.
6. Resident will ask family and friends to attend a community activity with him.

Chapter Four

Case Study

Vera

Vera is a 76-year-old female resident of Shady Pines, a 110-bed Nursing Home which is located in a rural area outside of Vera's hometown which has a population of approximately 10,000. She has lived at Shady Pines for 1 year. She has a primary diagnosis of diabetes mellitus, uses a wheelchair for mobility and needs assistance with ADL's. Her daughter lives locally but visits infrequently. Vera prefers to interact with staff one-to-one and usually refuses to leave her room for activities. She smokes cigarettes daily and visits the beauty parlor twice a month. She does attend Protestant Services in the nursing home once a week. She frequently watches her roommate's TV.

Comprehensive Therapeutic Recreation Assessment Summary

Resident: Vera Smith #: 402
Room #: 331 Date: 9/19/95

Summary of Functioning Levels

Physical:
Uses a wheelchair for mobility, has impaired range of motion, reduced endurance, and vertigo. Primary diagnosis of diabetes mellitus. Needs assistance with dressing, bathing, toileting, and transferring.

Mental:
Oriented to person, place and time, some mild short-term memory impairment. Follows directions. Short attention span.

Emotional:
Easily frustrated, reports feeling sad, frequent crying episodes observed by staff. Feels tired most of the time. Wishes she would die.

Social:
Has one daughter living locally who visits infrequently. Daughter feels too overworked and overwhelmed by Vera's problems to visit. Able to communicate. Dislikes group activities. Frequently refuses to leave room. Prefers one-to-one interaction with staff.

Financial:
Limited financial resources. Resident smokes cigarettes, and all of her monthly allowance is spent between smoking and beauty parlor.

Spiritual:

Believes in afterlife in heaven. She is Baptist and attends weekly Protestant services in the nursing home.

Occupational:

She worked in a garment factory most of her life and retired at 65 years of age.

LEISURE

Control:

External locus of control—she feels victimized by her health status and age.

Competence:

Says she's not good at anything anymore.

Attitudes:

Has a strong work ethic. Does not value leisure.

Playfulness:

Very little sense of humor or spontaneity.

Participation:

Attends weekly church service, visits beauty parlor twice a month. Receives one-to-one visits from activity staff. She frequently watches her roommate's TV.

Needs:

Companionship and escape.

Leisure Interests

Major Past Interests:

Sitting on the porch, going for rides in the car, going out to dinner, family get-togethers, watching TV, talking on the phone, sewing, gardening, and church activities.

Major Current Interests:

Church, TV, beauty parlor.

Comparison of Past and Present and Types:

Decrease in present interests compared to past. Vera says this is because she can no longer do the other things she enjoys. She has always disliked games and arts & crafts.

Leisure Constraints

Intraindividual Constraints

Physical:
Wheelchair mobility, reduced endurance, impaired ROM, vertigo, 1,200 calorie diabetic diet.

Environmental:
Limited financial resources.

Sensory:
None reported.

Extraindividual Constraints

Communication:
None reported.

Interpersonal:
Difficulty interacting intraindividually, extraindividually, aggregate, unilaterally, multilaterally and intragroup. Refuses to leave room frequently. Dislikes interacting with other residents.

Family:
Infrequent contact with daughter. Resident desires more frequent contact. Daughter uncomfortable visiting nursing home.

Behavioral:
None reported.

Interindividual Constraints

Emotional:
Reports feeling sad, frequent crying episodes observed, lack of interest in activities, tired.

Attitudes:
Strong work ethic. Does not value leisure. Low motivation. Lacks confidence in abilities.

Cognitive:
Short attention span. Mild short-term memory impairment.

Needs

Physical:
None unmet.

Safety and Trust:
Needs freedom to remain in room. Needs safe space. Needs to have control and choices.

Love and Belonging:
Desires one-to-one companionship. Dislikes being alone and in groups. Does not feel part of any group, except religious affiliation.

STRENGTHS	WEAKNESSES
strong religious affiliation	lacks feelings of competence
desires companionship	lacks feelings of control
past interests possible to adapt	lacks playfulness
strong work ethic	refuses participation
desires escape in leisure	refuses to leave room

Learning Opportunity

Directions: Prioritize *all* of Vera's problems/needs and strengths from your own therapeutic perspective. Evaluate each problem/need according to the criteria presented in Chapter Two.

PROBLEMS/NEEDS	STRENGTHS

Then answer the following questions:
1. Which problems/needs would you choose to address? Why?
2. Which ones would improve her quality of life the most? Why?
3. Which strengths would you choose to use to address the problems/needs? Why?

Compare your list with the Suggestions and Discussion that follow.

DISCUSSION

PROBLEMS/NEEDS	STRENGTHS
Diabetes mellitus	Has locally located daughter
Mobility and ADL impaired	Attends church
Refuses to leave room	Enjoys TV viewing
Smokes	Communicates needs and feelings
Easily frustrated	Interested in appearance
Feels sad and tired	Oriented times three
Limited financial resources	Follows directions
Poor self esteem	Enjoys one-to-one interactions
External locus of control	Strong work ethic
Little playfulness	Worked in garment industry most of life
Lack of interest	Enjoyed talking on phone in past
Short attention span	Interested in closer ties with family

Although each therapist might approach this case differently, the following suggestions serve as a guideline in goal planning. First, remember to build on Vera's strengths and interests. With these in mind the recreation therapist may choose to design an intervention that:

1. Internalizes Vera's locus of control.
2. Improves Vera's opportunities for companionship with her family.
3. Revitalizes the past leisure skills involved with using the telephone.
4. Helps Vera regain family contact and a sense of usefulness.

Suggested goals:

1. Vera will learn how to use the nursing home pay phone.
   - Vera will receive phone call instruction in her room three times during the first week of the plan.
   - Vera will accompany her therapist on a tour outside of her room three times to learn where the pay phone is located during the second week of the plan.
   - Vera will make herself a phone list and change holder to take to the phone.

2. Vera will leave her room to make calls on the pay phone in the hallway.
   - Vera will be accompanied by a nurses aide to telephone her therapist three times during the fourth week of the plan.
   - Vera will telephone her therapist independently three times during the fifth week of the plan.
3. Vera will independently arrange to do sewing/mending for her daughter's family.
   - Vera will independently call her daughter to chat during the sixth week of the plan.
   - Vera will call her daughter to offer to do mending and arrange for the daughter to bring the items to the nursing home.

It is hoped that this intervention will help Vera to feel useful and more able to control things that happen to her. She is building on the desire to have more contact with her daughter, the ability to sew/mend, and her past interest of talking on the phone. She is leaving her room independently, receiving positive one-to-one interactions, and structuring her own free time. Progress on these goals will significantly improve Vera's quality of life.

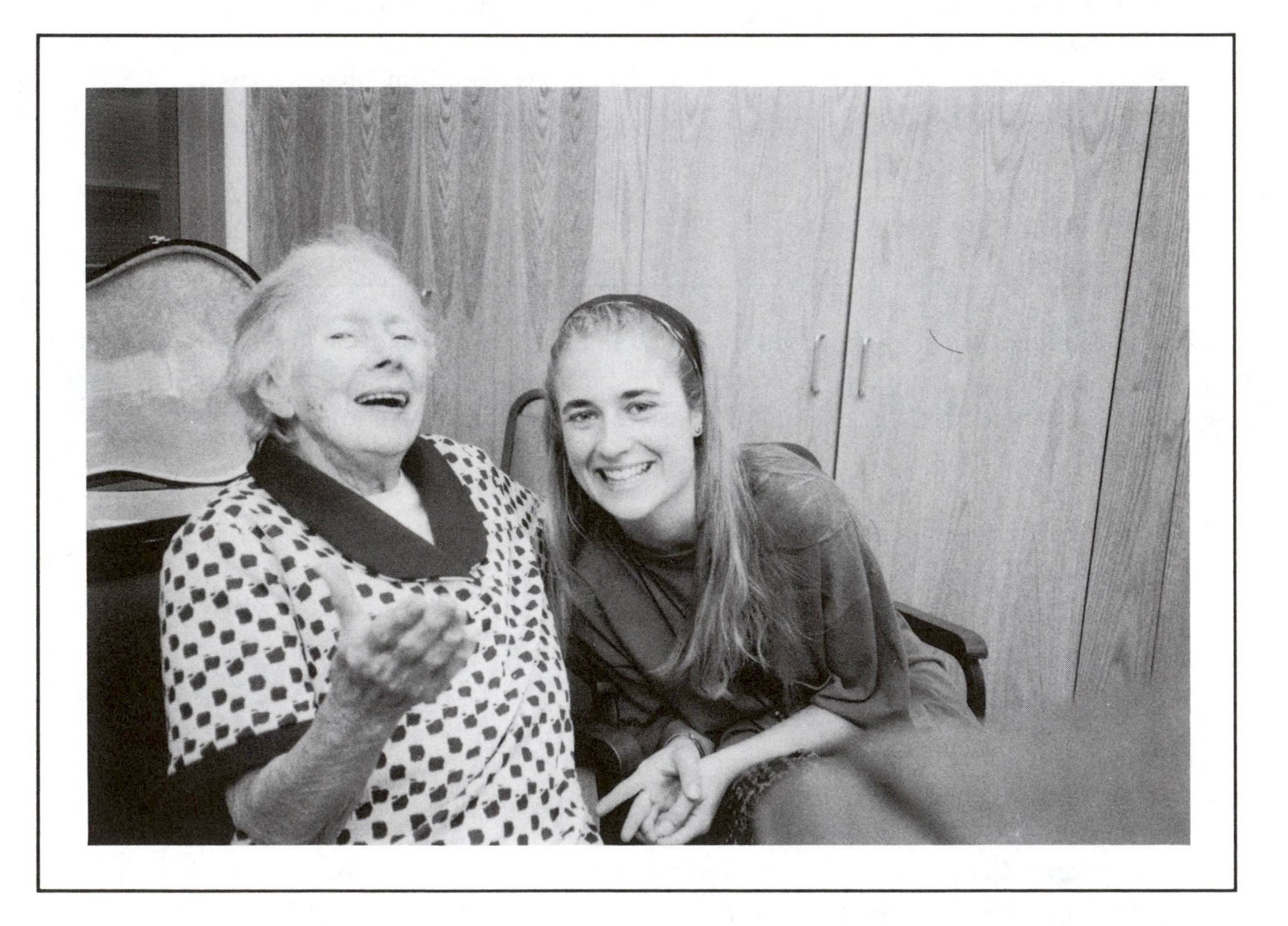

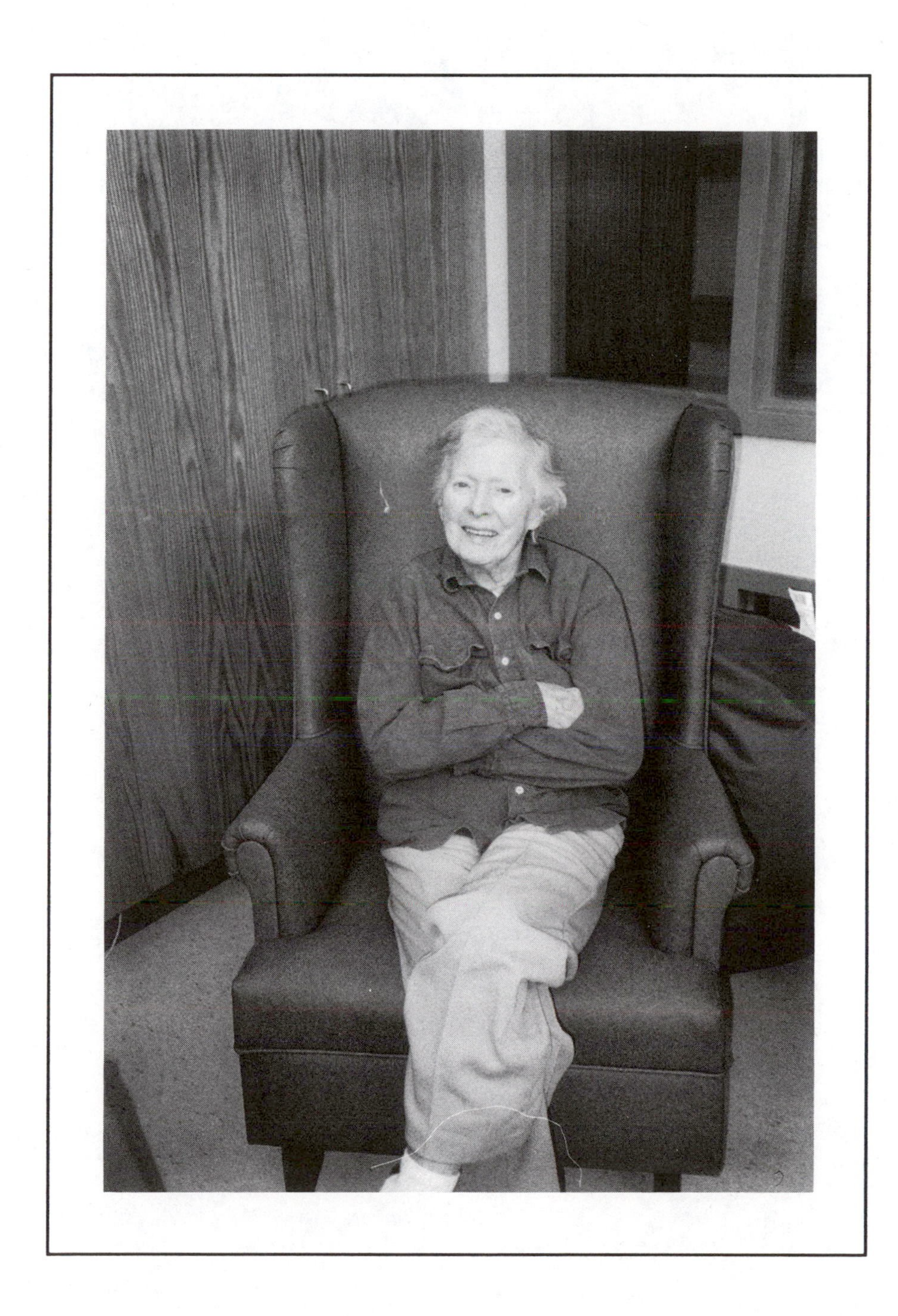

Chapter Five
Planning Interventions

Once a goal has been determined, the intervention can be planned. Usually the intervention is completed within a leisure activity that the resident likes. Care must be used in choosing an activity that will allow the goal to be reached. For instance, a popular goal in the nursing home is to increase social interaction with other residents. It would be best to choose an activity that by its nature requires the participants to communicate and interact with each other. Bingo, for example, does not require the participants to talk or interact with each other, so this would not be a good choice for this particular goal. Password, on the other hand, does require the participants to talk with each other, and therefore would be a good choice for this goal.

Activity analysis is the process by which individual activities are scrutinized to determine if they would be helpful in reaching a certain goal. Peterson and Gunn (1984), in their book *Therapeutic Recreation Program Design,* present a useful format for this process. Each area of an activity is investigated for its usefulness in meeting particular goals. Basically, the activity should be compared to the areas of assessment to see if they are compatible. For example, the various aspects of an activity should be broken down into separate sections: physical, social, mental, emotional, financial, environmental, and leisure aspects. These can then be examined to see if the activity's goals are compatible with the resident's goals.

Peterson and Gunn (1984) suggest the following questions should be answered for each activity considered:

Physical:

1. What is the primary body position required?
2. What parts of the body are required?
3. What types of movement does the activity require?
4. How much coordination is needed between parts and movements?
5. What are the primary senses required for the activity?
6. How much eye-hand coordination is needed?
7. How much strength is required?
8. How much speed is required?
9. How much endurance is needed?
10. How much flexibility is needed?

Social:

1. What type of social interaction pattern is primary to the activity?
2. How many participants does the activity require?
3. Does the nature of the activity encourage participants to communicate with each other?
4. Is the activity cooperative or competitive?
5. How much physical contact is necessary?
6. How structured is the activity?
7. What is the noise level?

Cognitive:

1. How many rules are there and are they complex?
2. How much immediate recall is necessary?
3. How much strategy does the activity require?
4. How much concentration is required?
5. Is it necessary to be able to read, write, spell, or use math?
6. How complex is scoring?
7. Must the participant be able to distinguish colors, size, objects, numbers, classes of objects, symbols, or do abstract thinking?
8. How many directions must the participant know? (left/right, up/down, etc.)

Emotional:

1. How many feelings may be expressed as part of the activity? (joy, guilt, pain, anger, fear, frustration)

Administrative:

1. What type of leadership is necessary? (supervision, teaching skills, etc.)
2. What equipment and facilities are needed?
3. What is the duration of the activity?
4. How many participants are necessary?

Leisure aspects should also be considered in addition to these presented by Peterson and Gunn (1984). Some suggestions are:

1. How much choice and control is available in the activity?
2. What is the attributional foundation of the activity? (luck, task difficulty, effort, ability)
3. How much playfulness is necessary? Possible?
4. What depth of involvement is necessary? Possible?
5. What level of creativity is necessary? Possible?
6. How much anxiety is inherent in the activity?
7. In what time frame is the activity centered? (past, present, future)
8. How much time and money are required to complete the activity?
9. Does the activity promote autonomy/independence?
10. How much fun/pleasure/humor is possible in the activity?
11. How much risk is involved?
12. Does the activity allow for active and passive participation?

Activity Adaptation

Nursing home activities have a long and rich history which includes many classic programs. The types of residents who now live in nursing homes have changed over the years. Residents are now sicker, both physically and mentally, and therefore have different programming needs. Traditional nursing home activities may not reach the resident who is physically very frail or severely cognitively impaired. The resident who is anxious or depressed is often considered inappropriate for traditional activities. These residents spend much of the day alone and isolated with few opportunities for meaningful involvement.

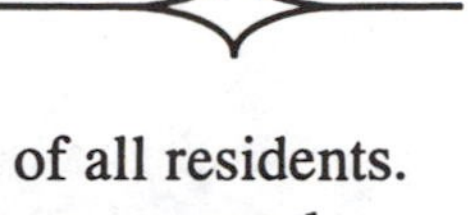

Activity analysis can help therapy staff adapt programs better meet the needs of all residents. The recreation therapist should identify the essential features of the activities that are currently offered. These features can give insight into the benefits of each program. Moreover, the analysis can be useful in modifying activities to make them more accessible and appropriate for the residents. The adaptations used should be minimal to allow the activity to be as similar to the original as possible.

The therapist should know the functioning levels and the interests of her residents from the TR assessment that was completed. She must now develop programs that match the residents' interests, needs and abilities. The therapist must then be able to adapt the activities without losing the essence of the endeavor.

"Rain Gutter Bocce League"

Many of the residents enjoyed playing croquet in the past. The nursing home did not have an adequate and safe lawn area for this activity, and very few residents were physically capable of playing the traditional form of the game. Managing a mallet and visually tracking the small wire targets were impossible for most.

The recreation therapist decided to try an adapted version of the game which was similar to bocce. The residents helped decorate an old sheet with bright colors and drew target areas which had point values. The sheet was placed on a patch of grass about 30 feet away. The corners were fixed by pushing large nails through them into the ground.

Croquet balls were used with a different color for each of the six resident-players. The idea was to toss or roll the ball to score on the sheet-target. The therapist soon discovered that some of the residents could not release the ball due to their arthritic joints. For those residents, a plastic rain gutter was used to assist the throw. From a sitting position, the rain gutter was lined up, and the ball was released. This adapted activity soon became so popular that an evening league was formed, with a team from each wing of the facility competing. Teams often included a nursing staff member as a coach, took on names for themselves, and sported colorful T-shirts for competition!

Normalization

Another important principle to consider in therapeutic programming is that of "normalization." Care must be taken when adapting activities so that residents are offered opportunities for a lifestyle that is as close to their norm as possible. The recreation therapist should try to normalize the daily schedule to match the routine of older adults. Not many older adults play table games at 9:30 in the morning. The day, the month, and the time of year programs are offered should also be normalized. How many community-dwelling older adults go to church on Tuesday at 6:30 in the evening?

All adaptations should also be age appropriate. Never use children's toys to meet an adaptation need for adults in the nursing home. For example, a teddy bear is not an age appropriate substitute for a family pet that was lost upon entry into the nursing home. Ask if most people this age who live in the community would be using this equipment? If the answer is no, it may not be

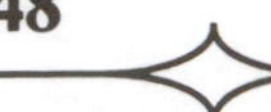

age appropriate. For example, is using crayons or blowing bubbles appropriate? Most older adults living in the community generally do not use either of these leisure materials of their own accord. Therefore, in most circumstances they would not be age appropriate in the nursing home. Aging is *not* returning to childhood, and it is never appropriate to use children's activities or materials in programming. To do so is a violation of the resident's right to be treated with dignity.

Normalize respect for the wishes of the individuals in your programs. Plan your programs with the input of the residents. Many nursing homes have resident planning committees, but these groups do not often include the more difficult-to-program residents. Early morning programs should be used to educate residents about daily events that might interest them, and then to listen to their suggestions.

Normalize the environment in which programs are offered. Try to do gardening programs outdoors. Do your cognitive therapy sessions in a stimulating environment. Cooking groups should meet in the kitchen or dining area. Teach leisure education skills in the environment in which they will be used. Use the local community as much as possible in your programming.

Planning for TR interventions, including activity analysis, adaptation, and normalization factors, must also take account of OBRA which requires that all nursing homes offer recreational activities which are therapeutic and not merely diversional.

OBRA Legislation and Empowerment

In 1977, Moss and Halamandaris wrote *Too Old, Too Sick, Too Bad* based on surveys of 1,373,465 occupants of 15,092 long-term care facilities. This book mirrored the simultaneous U.S. Senate investigation of the nursing home industry. It was disclosed that 80% of the nursing homes in the U.S. were profit oriented, and questioned the conflict of interest between profits and residents' welfare. Unlicensed and overworked staff was responsible for up to 90% of the resident care, and over 50% of these institutions were considered substandard. Residents who did not offer tips to their caretakers, or who were not on their favorites list, frequently went without baths, shaves, clean clothes, and sheets. They also did not receive assistance in toileting, being left to sit in urine and feces. Drugs were the main type of treatment for physical as well as mental impairments, and as many as 50% of medications were incorrectly dispensed. Residents who had behavioral problems were often physically or chemically restrained. As late as 1989, the Pennsylvania Division of Long-Term Care reported that 38% of residents nationwide were physically restrained (many states reported incident rates as high as 40 to 50%) and 27% of residents were receiving psychotropic drugs, most without a supporting psychiatric diagnosis. This survey revealed that as many as 50% of residents in some states were not being toileted. Clearly, quality care was not being given to residents of nursing homes.

In response to these conditions, the Health Care Finance Administration (HCFA) turned to the National Academy of Sciences for assistance. They commissioned the Institute of Medicine to conduct a study to determine how to improve quality of care in nursing homes. The results indicated that the focus of care should be quality of life, not medical treatment. HCFA accepted the results of the study and endorsed legislation to rectify the situation. The Omnibus Budget Reconciliation Act of 1987 (OBRA '87) was enacted on December 22, 1987 (Department of Health, Federal Register, 1989). HCFA's holiday present to the nursing home resident was a far reaching reorganization of Medicare and Medicaid certification requirements for long-term care.

The focus of the OBRA legislation is quality of life for the nursing home resident. This is accomplished through affirming the legal rights of residents concerning freedom of choice, dignity, self-determination, and freedom from restraints. Recreation is included as a component of the quality of life and three types of activity programming are to be included in every facility:

> Empowerment Activities: Activities which promote increased self-respect by providing opportunities for self-expression, personal responsibility, and choice.
>
> Maintenance Activities: Activities which provide a schedule of events that promote physical, cognitive, social, and emotional health.
>
> Supportive Activities: Activities which provide stimulation or solace to residents who cannot generally benefit from other types of activities. (Department of Health, Federal Register, 1989)

Myers (1990) and Waters and Goodman (1990) both proposed the concept of empowerment as a method of dealing with older adults which enables them to regain control over their lives. The authors use this method to overcome or avert feelings of helplessness in adults who have experienced many losses. Self-esteem and self-worth can be increased by empowering older adults to become self-determined. Empowerment can be accomplished by helping one to increase his or her level of independence, self-respect, and perceived freedom. Through education, adults can be taught decision-making skills and how to identify and maximize their choices. Empowerment activities are those activities which increase perceived freedom in leisure. Historically, most recreation programs in nursing homes have concentrated on maintenance and supportive activities. OBRA legislation has added the requirement for empowerment activities, but has not specifically named activities which meet these characteristics. To clarify these activities it is necessary to review empirical research on activities which may increase perceived freedom, control, and choice.

Program Planning and Empowerment

OBRA legislation was designed to minimize the effects of residing in an institution. Institutionalization has been thought to have many negative effects. Sommer and Osmond (1960-61) theorized that people residing in institutions had less ability to show independence in their actions and thoughts, less ability to retain cultural values and attitudes, the potential for increased psychological or physical decline, increased estrangement from the community, and a feeling of isolation from family and friends.

Individual choice of residents is frequently sacrificed for the efficiency of the institution. A study by Hulicka, Morganti and Cataldo (1975) found that older people residing in the community felt they had much more choice than those residing in a nursing facility. Often, residents of a nursing home have no choice in entering the facility. Ferrari (1962) asked 55 females how much choice they had in relocating to a nursing home. Almost one-third (31%) felt they had no choice. Only one of the women who felt she had no choice was alive 10 weeks later. Ferrari also compared two groups of nursing home admissions: one group who chose to enter the institution, and the other group whose families made the application for them. Eighty-six percent of those whose families made application died in the first month of residence in the institution compared to only 22% of the group who exercised free choice. Lack of perceived control in the aged may increase mortality rates. Seligman (1975) used these data to theorize that lack of control can lead to depression and then ultimately to death in older people.

Many potential losses face aging adults in varying degrees: loss of job, spouse, mobility, health, income, financial security, family, friends, cognitive abilities, and physical endurance. Adaptation to these losses is the principle challenge of aging (Teague, 1980). An additional loss experienced by many older adults is loss of control over many aspects of their own lives. This happens in a number of ways. The scout helping the old woman across the street is imbedded in society's mind. This bias permeates attitudes toward the elderly. It is at the root of the loss of control experienced in the healthcare system, in community services provided for older adults, and in interpersonal and family relationships with older adults. Society views older people, women especially, as being too old to think for themselves. Aging is often equated with senility, paving the way for the young to step in and take control. This happens at a time when most older people are feeling "entitled to do what pleases and satisfies... [themselves], to slow down, to let go the strain of former obligations, to express...thoughts and feelings more strongly than ever before" (Doress & Siegal, 1987). Many older adults are not afforded the opportunity to do that which they desire because of the societal biases of age and sex.

The end result of these various kinds of loss of control is that the older adult often ends up in an environment which constrains self-determination (MacNeil & Teague, 1987). Self-determination is a basic human right, and when people lose this right, there are consequences such as low self-esteem, diminished self-concept, feelings of hopelessness, depression, and helplessness (Howe-Murphy & Charboneau, 1987, p. 112). Control over the environment is positively correlated with mental and physical health (Langer & Rodin, 1976; Shulz, 1976). Therefore, one of the major mental and physical health concerns of older adults is that they remain in control over their surroundings, their personal lives, and their leisure (MacNeil & Teague, 1987). Iso-Ahola (1980) wrote, "the main task of the [recreation] therapist is to increase the patients' perceived control and mastery over the environment and to prevent them from inferring helplessness" (p. 323). According to Peterson and Gunn (1984) control by the individual should be built into therapeutic recreation programs. The authors suggest that participants be able to choose the activity, choose voluntarily to participate, and control their own involvement in the activity. They sight a "high degree of freedom and participant control" as being essential to all therapeutic programming (p. 46). Frye and Peters (1972) present a continuum from authority by the recreation leader to freedom of choice by the participant as the goal in the therapeutic relationship. Howe-Murphy and Charboneau (1987) state that the main outcome of a helper and client relationship should be the "transfer of authority for decision making from the helper to the client" (p. 56).

Bengtson (1973) believed that providing total care for individuals in a nursing home without providing them a right to make choices, is just as bad as providing no care at all. Langer and Rodin (1976) investigated the effects of lack of choice and control by conducting an experiment with 91 residents of a nursing home. They divided them into two groups. One group was told that they were responsible for themselves, while the other group was told that the staff was responsible for all residents. The choice group was allowed to make decisions on activities, room decor, and other personal items, while the no-choice group was not allowed to make decisions. Both groups were tested before, and three weeks following the intervention, for the following characteristics:

happiness, activeness, and alertness. Results showed that the choice group had increased in all three categories, while the no choice group did not. Nurses were asked to rate both groups, and 93% of the choice group was rated to have progressed, while 71% of the no choice group was rated to have declined in overall status. Results also confirmed that increased choices of activities increased the number of activities attended by the residents. The choice group also attended more active programs, while the no choice group attended more passive ones.

Rodin and Langer (1977) extended the previous study by observing the same subjects over an 18-month period. The choice group maintained or increased their health ratings during this time, while the no-choice group continued a significant decline in health status. The mortality rates for both groups were compared, and the choice group's rate was 15% compared to a 30% rate for the no-choice group. The study controlled for differences in beginning health status of subjects. These long-range data confirmed that increased choice lowers mortality rates and improves, or at least maintains, health status. Jeffares (1986) established that freedom of choice was one of the main factors in morale and happiness in elderly residents living in public housing.

One of the areas in which control is lost in the nursing home is in social contacts with others. Schulz (1976) investigated the effects of control over social interaction on health status, zest for life, hope, and future orientation. Forty-two residents of a retirement home (36 women and 6 men), with an age range between 67 and 96 years, were divided into four groups. The first group was a control visitor group, which was allowed to choose the frequency and duration of visits from a college student over a 2-month period. The second group was a predicted visitor group, which was informed of the frequency and duration of the visits but had no control in this determination. The third group was a random visitor group, which received unscheduled random visits from the students. The fourth group was not visited by the students. After the treatment, the activities director who was a long-time former nurse at the facility was asked to rate the subjects on a health status scale and a zest for life scale. The activity director knew nothing about the experiment and therefore was not aware in which group each subject participated. Subjects also completed four questionnaires prior to and following treatment. The questionnaires were titled "Activities," "My Usual Day," "Future Diary," and "The Wohlford Hope Scale." An additional three scales were administered after treatment. These scales were used to gather information on the subject's background and stay at the home, information about the visitor program, and information on their happiness, health status, and usefulness. The results indicated that the residents who could predict or control visits were rated to be more healthy and were taking less medication than those who received random visits or no visits at all. Physically, the predict and control subjects maintained their health status, while the random and no visit groups declined. Psychologically, the control and predict groups improved their status while the random and no visit groups declined on ratings of zest for life, hope, and future orientation. The control and predict groups were more active than the other groups. There were no significant differences between the control and predict groups in the measures used.

To test the long-term effects of control over social interaction on health status, Shulz and Hanusa (1978) conducted a follow-up study with the same groups as above at 24, 30, and 42 month intervals following the original period of visitation. This investigation indicated that the benefits gained by the control and predicted groups were temporary, since their physical and psychological health status returned to the level of the other two groups by the end of the study (3.5 years). Thus, choice and control intervention must be consistent and ongoing to be effective.

The benefits of having control over social interaction with other people in the environment also can be found when control is exercised over objects in the environment. Banzinger and Roush (1983) conducted experiments on the relationship between having control over an object in the environment, and a resident's interpersonal and physical activity level and life satisfaction. Forty nursing home residents ranging in age from 57 to 98 participated in the study. They were divided into three groups. One group was given the opportunity to have a bird feeder to care for on their own, and was given a message which indicated that they were responsible for the bird feeder. They had the opportunity to choose to participate in the program and to choose which type of bird feeder they would place in their window. The second group was also given a bird feeder, but received a message that indicated they were not responsible for the feeder but dependent on others to care for it. The third group did not receive a bird feeder or a message. The group which was chosen to control the bird feeders was judged by staff to have higher levels of involvement and attendance at activities than the other two groups. Self-report questionnaires showed that the bird feeder control group had higher levels of control, happiness, activity, and life satisfaction than the other two groups. Having a sense of control over one's environment can increase participation in recreation programs, and overall life satisfaction.

Religious and spiritual participation also offers the resident many opportunities for choice and increased control over life. Baack (1985) studied 198 seniors over age 60 who were involved in community and religious recreation programs and identified religious involvement as a predictor of perceived freedom in leisure.

When working with institutionalized older adults, recreation staff should give responsibility of choice to the resident. Robertson (1988) developed a continuum of choice and intervention for the therapeutic recreation professional working with nursing home residents where residents progress from intervention by the specialist to total choice by the resident. Peterson and Gunn's (1984) therapeutic recreation service model also moves from intervention by the therapist to independent choice by the client. Leisure education can be a method of increasing resident's skills in identifying and making choices in leisure. Rodin (1983) found that residents who received training in making choices felt more in control and were more active than other groups that did not receive training.

People who choose their activity will participate longer in that activity. Realon, Favell, and Lowerre (1990) found that adults with severe handicaps interacted longer during leisure pursuits which were chosen freely by the individual, as opposed to those selected for the individual by the staff. Parsons, Reid, Reynolds, and Bumgarner (1990) found that if the subjects chose their activity, they attended to it longer than if the task was assigned.

Residents of nursing homes should be involved in planning as well as choosing their own recreation programs. Mannell, Zuzanek, and Larson (1988) examined the leisure choices of 92 retired adults who reflected normal adult psychological patterns. The authors discovered that in groups where activities were freely chosen by the subjects there was higher positive affect, more concentration, and less feelings of tension, than in groups where activities were assigned. Involving residents in programming may be time consuming, but it has beneficial effects for the participants.

Freedom of choice is paramount to feelings of satisfaction in retirement. Russell (1984) found that retirement satisfaction is greater when residents feel high levels of choice and control. Life satisfaction could be increased by increasing residents' choice and control over the environment and others in the environment.

There is little research on specific activities and the level of perceived freedom felt by participants. Gottesman and Bourstom (1974) investigated time use of nursing home residents and found that 56% of their time is spent in passive activities. These are defined as doing nothing, resting, waiting, sitting, or thinking.

Voelkl (1989) also investigated time use by nursing home residents and found that 35% of their time was spent in passive activities. This accounted for the largest chunk of time in the day. She also found that most time is spent in solitude (63%) and in their own rooms (85%). She investigated the degree of control felt by the residents in these various activities. High levels of control were experienced by the residents when they were with others, especially staff and visitors, and when engaged in an independent activity. The residents did not feel in control when alone, when engaging in passive activities, when eating, when watching television, or when with other residents of the nursing home.

"The espoused goal of nursing homes is often summarized in terms of the three R's: to restore, rehabilitate and return to the community." (Teague, MacNeil, & Hitzhusen, 1982. p. 258). OBRA '87 mandates this approach to nursing quality care in the nursing home is empowering home care: an important part of the provision of the resident with as much choice and control as possible. Bowker (1982) states that "providing residents with opportunities for choice and responsibility seems to have many beneficial results" on their quality of life (p. 11). It is the responsibility of the therapeutic recreation staff to provide these opportunities for empowerment and to keep these principles in mind when planning interventions and activities.

Martin and Smith (1993) offer the following guidelines to enhance residents' sense of control and freedom through recreation:

1. Assess and monitor the residents' perceptions of control.
2. Provide optimal levels of choice whenever possible with at least two and not more than six options.
3. Utilize leisure education activities to facilitate choice making.
4. Involve residents in the recreation activity planning process. Give them as much control as possible over their own programs.
5. Provide activities based on individual needs and preferences. Do not simply fit residents into an existing activity schedule. Instead, fit the schedule to the residents' interests.
6. Reduce or eliminate barriers to participation.
7. Ensure that activities are age-appropriate.
8. Normalize activities.
9. Provide opportunities for social interaction.
10. Include opportunities for spiritual development.
11. Emphasize active participation in planning.

Community Integration

Maslow (1968) writes that one of people's basic needs is to feel love and to belong. Everyone needs to feel connected as part of at least one group. Jean Baker Miller (1976), in her book *Toward a New Psychology of Women,* talks about women developing and growing in "connection" with others. It may be particularly important therefore, for women especially, to retain a sense of connection with the community while residing in the nursing home. Extra effort should be made to sustain any existing connections to organizations or groups in the community when older adults enter the nursing home. This can be done in two ways. First, and easiest, bring the community into the nursing home. This can be done through inviting community organizations to perform, or provide services inside the nursing facility, or attend events sponsored by and in the nursing home, such as lectures and concerts. Second, residents should have the opportunity to go out into the community at least once a month, even if it is only for an automobile ride around a familiar neighborhood. Other popular events are concerts, religious services, and dining out at local restaurants. Trips can be made to state parks, farms, and other local attractions. The adopt-a-grandparent program is an example of a successful community link with young people. It is very important that the resident have the opportunity to retain her sense of connection with her community.

Section Three

Implementation

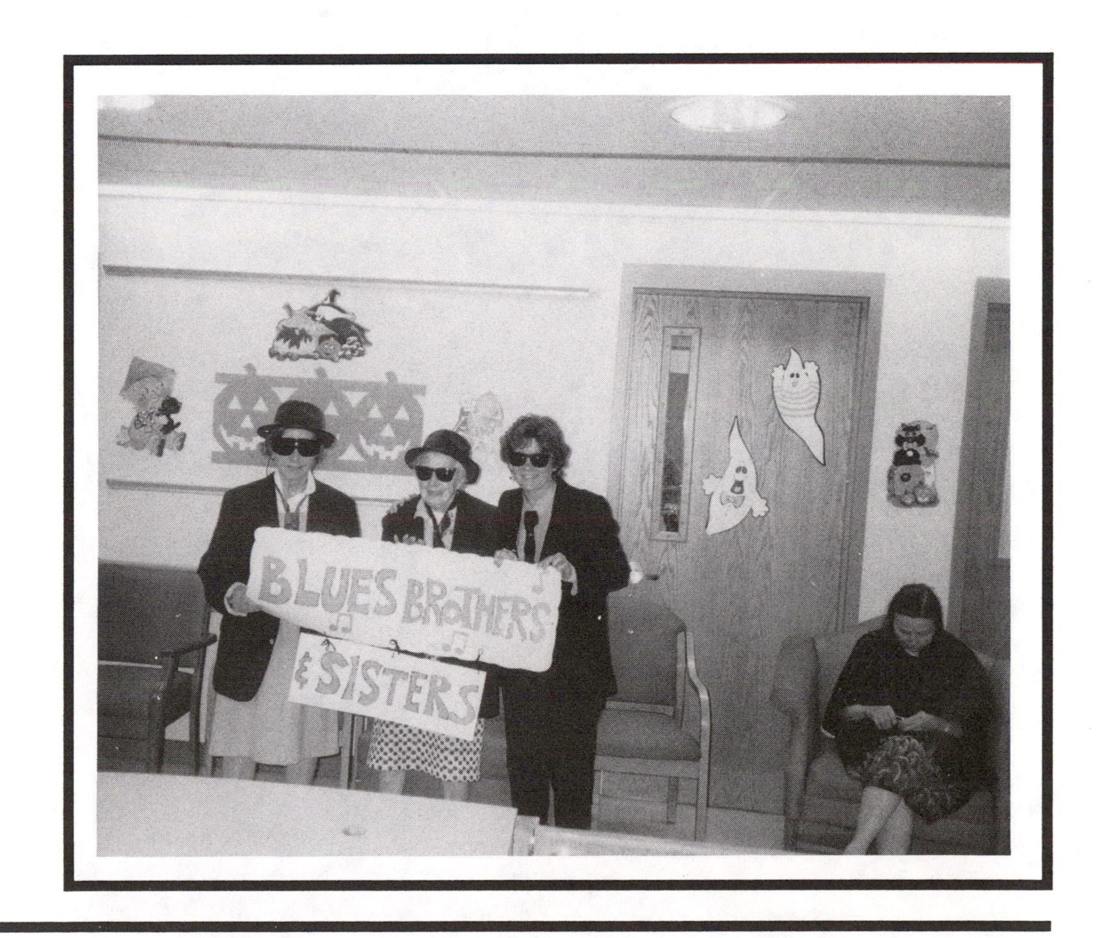

Chapter Six
Therapeutic Relationships

Empowerment "is a process by which individuals gain mastery and control over their lives, and a critical understanding of their environment" (Zimmerman, Israel, Shulz, & Checkoway, 1992). This intervention is widely used in feminist therapy to help women take control of their lives and destiny. It is an intervention which could be applied in the nursing home setting to help residents regain or maintain self-determination.

Psychotherapy carries many negative stereotypes and connotations for individuals who are older; however, empowerment, a therapeutic intervention based on the humanistic psychology of Maslow and Rogers, is a method that can be used by all staff and all disciplines. Self-determination or perceived freedom is a crucial component of both leisure and empowerment. Since perceived freedom is the most important component of the leisure experience (Neulinger, 1974), leisure or recreation is an area of nursing home life that is particularly well-suited to the intervention of empowerment.

Murphy (1975) has written that leisure services embrace a humanistic view of human nature and intervention. Empowerment through therapeutic recreation seems a natural extension of these tenants. One method of intervention which could be useful in empowerment in the nursing home is the technique of play therapy espoused by Virginia Axline (1969). Her technique was originally developed for use with children, but could be adapted for use with older adults in the nursing home. Because of concerns for age-appropriate terminology when working with older adults, play therapy in this setting will be referred to as "leisure empowerment."

The primary aspect of empowerment through leisure empowerment is that it occurs in the relationship between therapist and resident. The empowering relationship that clears the way for growth is an emotionally safe environment in which the resident is able to explore characteristics of himself or herself (Maslow, 1968). Carl Rogers (1961) described this relationship in detail. The helping relationship can be one-to-one or group centered. The most important factors that determine the quality of this relationship are the attitudes and feelings of the helper (Rogers, 1961). Rogers believed that these attitudes are far more important than procedures, techniques, or knowledge. The following are attitudes which Rogers outlines for effective and empowering relationships. One important note: not only is it important for the staff to act in the following ways, but it is important for the residents to perceive these attitudes as well. In other words, the staff's actions and the residents' perceptions must agree (Rogers, 1957). It is a good idea to monitor those perceptions by asking residents for feedback on a regular basis.

Staff should be trustworthy, dependable, and consistent (Rogers, 1961). They should keep promises and appointments and be on time. Staff should never promise anything that they cannot deliver. Confidentiality and respect for resident's dignity are essential. No information or "cute stories" should be shared with other staff, unless it is absolutely necessary, and *never* for the entertainment purpose of staff. Trust is developed between the helper and the resident over time, and is an ongoing process (Johnson, 1981).

Staff behavior should be congruent (Rogers, 1961). The staff's attitudes and feelings must match their actions and words. The staff must be honest and genuine. Genuineness means being oneself without being phony or playing a role (Cormier & Cormier, 1985). For example, if a staff member is angry with a resident but tries to instead act as though nothing is wrong, the resident will sense this. This mismatch between feelings and communication will destroy any trust that has been built. One must be aware of one's feelings at all times and be sure that communications are congruent. Interventions that manipulate residents without their consent, such as behavior modification, should not be used. "In Skinner's thinking, a man must relinquish his beliefs in freedom and self-determination and come to accept the fact that he is controlled by forces outside himself" (Lefcourt, 1982, p. 2). Behavior modification is incompatible with empowerment unless a self-control technique is used. In this type of behavior modification the resident not only consents to the intervention, but also monitors her or his own behavior and takes rewards for behavior that she or he determines as desirable (Cormier & Cormier, 1985).

Residents should be viewed in a positive way and shown "attitudes of warmth, caring, liking, interest, [and] respect" (Rogers, 1961 p. 52). Impersonal professional aloofness is not a substitute for real caring. It will soon be detected by the resident. Warmth is an important ingredient in the helping relationship (Goldstein, 1980). Nonverbal behaviors are important expressions of warmth (Johnson, 1981). For example, a soft, soothing tone of voice, smiling, relaxed posture, appropriate eye contact, and touch communicate warmth. Gazda et al. (1984, p. 111) suggest asking the following questions when using touch with clients:

1. How does the other person perceive this? Is it seen as genuine or as a superficial technique?
2. Is the other person uncomfortable?
3. Am I interested in the person or in touching the person? Whom is it for—me, the other person, or is it to impress those who observe?

Find something to prize in each and every resident. By focusing on strengths, people can be viewed in a positive manner. Most characteristics can be viewed as strengths. Characteristics commonly viewed as weaknesses by society could be reframed and considered as strengths. This is done by looking at the purpose that the characteristic serves, and by viewing it as a method (that was learned) of meeting a particular need.

For example, Mary is an individual who is described by the medical staff as being a hypochondriac. She has complained of a pain in her hip. Many tests have been done and nothing can be found to be causing her pain. In leisure empowerment, Mary's hip pain could be viewed as a method that she learned to get attention from the medical staff. It would not be viewed as manipulative, but as a legitimate means learned to meet her needs for attention and social interaction. In fact, Mary's actions would be seen as a strength in that she was ingenious enough to find a way to get her needs met. Alternative methods of meeting these needs could be proposed and tried within the security of the therapeutic relationship, and then Mary could choose which methods she feels work best for her. In using this approach, change cannot be the mandated outcome. The staff must be willing to defer to the needs and desires of the resident. If Mary chooses to continue using her hip pain to gain attention from the staff, her decision must be accepted.

It would be contrary to this theoretical framework to institute a behavior modification program to reduce positive reinforcement from Mary's contact with staff. This would be denying her the freedom to meet her needs in a manner which she chooses.

Staff should view residents as innately good, not evil (Maslow, 1968). This is a philosophical orientation to human nature. Humanistic philosophies view individuals as capable of knowing what they need and the best way to meet that need. Residents should guide the assessment and goal setting process. Person-centeredness is a term that describes this attitude. It means that individuals are treated as persons, not as diseases or disabilities.

This attitude is demonstrated by the use of person-first terminology (Dattilo & Smith, 1990). Instead of referring to individuals as "diabetics," "amputees," or "wheelchair-bound," they are called "an individual with diabetes," "a person who has an amputation," or "individuals who use wheelchairs." This terminology should always be used when speaking to or about individuals with disabilities, and when writing in the medical chart. Individuals do not become their disabilities unless they are treated like a disability. Appreciation of the individuality and uniqueness of each person must guide therapeutic intervention.

Recognize the staff as separate persons with separate needs, feelings, and opinions (Rogers, 1961). This is a boundary issue. The staff member must not become enmeshed in the relationship, but retain a sense of self in interaction. For example, a recreation therapist may empathetically feel sadness with the loss of a resident's spouse, but must recognize that the sadness "belongs" to the resident, not the therapist. Also, the staff member may have different values, ideas, and morals than residents. This must be accepted comfortably. Residents should not be persuaded to adopt the staff's views.

Allow the resident the freedom to be who he or she is (Rogers, 1961). This means accepting the resident's right of self-determination and individuality. The resident knows what is best for herself or himself. Residents should not be cajoled into following advice or coerced into attending activities when they feel that they really would rather not. This is respecting the boundaries of the resident. This also means not judging or evaluating the resident's feelings, needs, or actions, but simply accepting them. Offer choices as much as possible. Since too many alternatives may be overwhelming, it is best to provide only two to six alternatives when asking for a choice (Aasen, 1987). If a resident makes a choice, staff should always abide by it and not take away the opportunity after the choice has been made.

The staff empathetically enters the resident's world (Rogers, 1961). They try to feel and see things as the resident does to better understand her or him. This information can then be reflected back to the resident, to check accuracy, to communicate understanding, and to give the resident the opportunity to understand herself or himself. Individualize programming so that each resident's needs are met. Use interest finders to help residents choose individual and group activities in the leisure therapy room. Families and volunteers can be used to provide some of these diverse opportunities. Families may have a particular piece of equipment, or a favorite instrument that a resident especially enjoys, and might be willing to loan it to the facility. Instead of fitting residents into a preplanned recreation schedule, leisure therapy allows programming to fit the individual interests and needs of residents. Activities included in the leisure therapy experience should be planned by residents, not for residents.

Accept the resident unconditionally and totally (Rogers, 1961). Silence following a shocking revelation by the resident communicates disapproval. So do many nonverbal actions such as frowning or surprise. Unconditional positive regard is an attitude which must be the guiding force of the helper. Positive regard must be unconditional in that it is not dependent on any action by the resident. This is shown through a nonjudgmental attitude no matter what the resident does. All feelings, thoughts, and behaviors are accepted as something important to the resident. Positive regard is neither approval nor disapproval, but acceptance. Anger and grief are emotions that many people have difficulty accepting. Emotional space must be made for these difficult feelings as well as for happy ones.

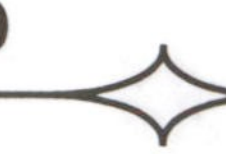

The staff must be sensitive, not threatening (Rogers, 1961). The resident will then feel safe enough to focus on her or his own threatening feelings (fear) from within. For example, Bill, a resident at Shady Pines Nursing Home, wishes he could learn to shoot pool. The TR specialist has won many competitions and awards in pool, and frequently boasts about his skill. Bill may feel threatened by the TR specialist's "expertise" in playing pool and probably will not feel safe enough to tell Bill about the time he totally embarrassed himself when trying to learn to play the game. He may feel foolish about asking questions, and sharing his feelings of incompetence and fears with the specialist. Instead, Bill is afraid to expose his feelings of vulnerability, and simply says he is not interested in playing pool.

Group participation can be threatening for many individuals. To make it nonthreatening, ground rules must be established. The resident must be able to start and stop participation when she or he feels like it. At the beginning of each group, residents should be reminded that they may choose not to participate at any time, and a sign should be agreed upon for passing a turn. It is often just as threatening to ask to pass as to participate, so a sign, like raising a hand in front of the face, is a less threatening way to pass. Residents can be encouraged to participate by reminding them that participation is challenging and can be stressful at times, but that it is rewarding to take the chance to participate.

Never force participation, but encourage and ask for it, i.e., "Please share your feelings with us." However, if the resident asks to pass or makes the pass sign, no further coaxing should be done. Accept the decision supportingly. Each resident taking a turn, or going around a circle is a good way to make sure that each resident has the opportunity to participate, but can be anxiety provoking for the resident. It is better to ask for volunteers so that residents who are less stressed about group participation can participate first, and then others can join in when they feel ready. Ample time should always be allowed for individuals to speak up. Supportive encouragement can be provided for residents who are unsure of themselves. At the end, specific residents who have not volunteered can be asked if they have anything to add. This gives them maximum time to get up courage to participate instead of being arbitrarily first or second by virtue of position in the circle.

The staff should free the residents from external evaluation (Rogers, 1961). What is important is the resident's evaluation, not what others think. Refrain from passing judgments. Underlying messages are very clear when saying things like, "That's good" or "You could do better" (that was bad). Instead, ask what the resident feels and reinforce or explore those feelings. Assessments frequently reflect the "expert's" opinion. In the empowerment process it is the resident's assessment of herself or himself that is important. The therapeutic leisure specialist is not considered an expert who assesses and diagnoses, but an equal human being who provides an emotionally safe environment (relationship) in which the resident feels comfortable exploring and identifying constraints and barriers to the leisure experience. Similarly, the resident should be encouraged to choose goals and evaluate progress. The therapeutic recreation specialist then charts this information using phrases like, "The resident feels .... The resident says it is important to her to ...." This does not mean that the therapist has no input, but that the resident's input is primary. When using a diagnostic tool, such as the leisure diagnostic battery, the results should be presented to the resident as a piece of information for her or him to evaluate and comment on. These comments should then be charted.

Focus on the present experience (Rogers, 1961). Do not be bound by the past or the future. If a resident does not swim because he or she never learned as a child, do not rule out the option of learning it in the present. The past is past. The future is uncertain. The resident who is always worrying "what if..." can be encouraged to focus on what is happening now. Staff can try to engage the resident in fully experiencing the present moment. This can be done by focusing on sensory experiences. Staff can ask, "How does that feel? (look, sound, taste, smell)." A resident who says that she or he was never any good at something can be reminded, "That was then, what about now?"

Present focus is particularly important in leisure, since the peak leisure experience, or flow experience is characterized by total involvement in the task at hand (Csikszentmihalyi, 1975). This is difficult for many people. There are times when reminiscing is a viable and beneficial task, but it should not be the overriding focus of the recreation program or a resident's life. Individuals are living in the present moment and can benefit from experiencing life in the present (Rogers, 1961). Certainly there is a sense of accomplishment to be felt when reviewing one's life, but to be limited to life in the past is to deny what life a resident has in the present and future. This leads to what is called a social death, where people, though living, are treated as though their lives are over (Cassell, 1974). Life is not over until it is over, and much satisfaction can be gained in living life to the end. As with most things, a balance between a healthy appreciation for the past and experiencing life in the future seems to be an even compromise.

Chapter Seven
The Adult Leisure Empowerment Environment

The Adult Leisure Empowerment Environment

The following guidelines for the physical environment of leisure empowerment are taken and adapted from Axline (1969). The optimal situation is to have a room dedicated to the leisure empowerment experience. However, in working one-to-one with residents who do not leave their beds or rooms, the leisure environment can be mobilized using a rolling cart containing appropriate materials for the individual residents. Likewise, day rooms can be transformed into a leisure empowerment environment permanently or on a rotating basis to share available resources in different sections of the nursing home. The following suggestions can be adapted to fit individual space and budgetary constraints of the facility. The room should be large enough to accommodate 10 to 15 residents who use standard wheelchairs. Residents should be able to move freely about the room with adequate maneuvering space between chairs and other furniture. Low shelves are useful for storing and displaying leisure materials. All shelves should be able to be viewed and seen easily from a wheelchair. There should be several tables in the room. One table should be large enough to accommodate group activity and should be round. Others should be able to provide individual work space, or dyad space. These can be round or square. All tables should be high enough to allow individuals in wheelchairs to sit adjacent to the table. Wheelchair arms should fit below the table. The room should be brightly colored and well-lighted. Daylight or simulated daylight fixtures are preferable. All surfaces in the room should be easily cleaned. Floors should be tile or vinyl. Colors should be as light and bright as possible. A sink in the room would be optimal, but not an absolute necessity. All decor should be age-appropriate, as should all materials. Under *no* circumstances should children's toys be used. It is important that the room being used for the leisure empowerment session be clearly designated as such, and not double as a staff break room during therapy sessions.

The materials presented for use in the room are suggestions. Therapeutic recreation specialists should feel free to try new and different items which meet the individual interests of the residents being served. It is suggested that materials be placed in baskets with handles. These baskets are then placed on the shelves. This would allow easy transportation of the materials by individuals using wheelchairs and walkers. Of course, small items such as a deck of cards need not be in a basket. However, if poker chips are available for use with the cards, then both could be placed in a basket for convenience. Likewise, score pads and pencils might be added to this basket to provide for flexibility of use. Similar materials should be grouped together, and areas of the room could be designated for specific use, such as exercise equipment, art materials, and musical area.

All materials should be age-appropriate. Staff should be creative in selecting items for the leisure environment. Resident input should be encouraged. Materials can be added or retired as usage indicates. Residents may request additional items after using the room. Staff should always include materials requested by the residents. Possible materials are listed in Figure 7.1, page 64. It is suggested that separate rooms, materials, and times be used in programming the leisure empowerment sessions for residents of differing cognitive abilities. The materials listed are primarily for residents of average cognitive ability. Some of these materials may be adaptable for residents who have cognitive impairments. Many companies manufacture and distribute activity materials designed for residents with dementia, and these materials should be included in leisure empowerment sessions with these adults. Never use age inappropriate materials with any adults, regardless of cognitive abilities.

Figure 7.1 Suggested Basic Materials For Leisure Empowerment

Art Materials	Music Resources	Exercise Resources
Acrylic Paints	Portable Keyboard	Exercise Bike
Brushes	Headphones	Treadmill
Canvas Tablets	Stereo/Tape Player	Stair Stepper
Sketching Supplies	Collection of Music	Rowing Machine
Clay	Rhythm Instruments	Weights
Craft Supplies	Songbooks	Mats
Woodworking	Various Drums	Air Mattress

Sports	Games	Other
Nerf Basketball	Rubber Tipped Darts	Sand Tray
Putting Green	Cards	Puzzles
Shuffleboard and Box	Jenga	Teaser Puzzles
Bocce Ball	Bandu	Trains
Horseshoes	Board Games	Remote Control Jeeps and Sand Track
Adapted Croquet	Checkers/Chess	Punching Bag
Volleyball/Badminton	Pinball	Ham Radio/CB
Pool	Ring Toss	Pets
Football	Trivia Games	Gardening
Table Tennis		Birdwatching
		Kites
		Flowers for Arranging

Leisure Empowerment Procedures

The following procedures are outlined by Axline (1969) for play therapy and are adapted for leisure empowerment with nursing home residents. Individual residents can be brought to the leisure empowerment room for one-to-one work, but the majority of interventions will take place in a group setting due to time and staffing constraints of the nursing home. Residents are invited to the leisure room as space and time permits. It is suggested that at least one session per week be available to each resident in the group setting, while two would be preferable. Optimally, the

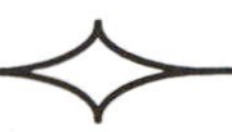

leisure empowerment room would be available to all residents at all times, but staff and budgetary constraints will prohibit this in most facilities.

The smaller the group, the more individual attention will be available to residents. The maximum group number should be about 15. Residents are encouraged to explore the room and activities offered on their own. At the beginning of each session, they should be reminded that this time is theirs to use as they please. Basic ground rules should be established. Residents may use anything in the room as they see fit. They should be asked to return items to the shelf when they are finished so that all residents may share the use of items as they wish. Materials should not be removed from the room, but if residents express such a desire, staff should make an effort to secure an additional item for use by the resident on her or his own.

Residents may interact with the materials individually or in groups. This decision should be left to the individual residents. No resident should be forced to do anything he or she does not want to do. The time spent in the leisure empowerment setting should be the resident's own. If the resident wants to sit and do nothing, it is permissible. The key element is freedom of choice. As much as possible, residents should be allowed to stay as long as they wish, or leave when they want. This freedom fosters the resident's sense of control, perceived competence, and self-esteem (Shary & Iso-Ahola, 1989). It should be noted that residents who do not regularly participate on their own in the leisure therapy group session may need to have individual 30-minute sessions with the therapist until such time as participation becomes spontaneous in the group situation.

In the group setting, several social interaction patterns may be observed. Avedon (1974) has identified eight interaction patterns of activities (see also Figure 2.1). These are as follows:

1. Intraindividual: "Action taking place within the mind of a person or action involving the mind and a part of the body, but requiring no contact with another person or external object" (p. 163). Examples: daydreaming, thinking, or imagery.
2. Extraindividual: "Action directed by a person toward an object in the environment, requiring no contact with another person" (p. 164). Examples: gardening, bird watching/feeding, and cooking.
3. Aggregate: "Action directed by a person toward an object in the environment while in the company of other persons who are also directing action toward objects in the environment. Action is not directed toward one another, and no interaction between participants is required or necessary" (p. 165). Examples: bingo, crafts, and entertainment programs.
4. Interindividual: "Action of a competitive nature directed by one person toward another." (p. 166). Examples: tennis, table tennis, chess, and any one-to-one sport.
5. Unilateral: "Action of a competitive nature among three or more persons, one of whom is an antagonist or it" (p. 167). Example: tag, and hide and seek. Few adult games fit this pattern.
6. Multilateral: "Action of a competitive nature among three or more persons, with no one person as an antagonist" (p. 168). Examples: poker, Scrabble, many board games.
7. Intragroup: "Action of a cooperative nature by two or more persons intent upon reaching a mutual goal. Action requires positive verbal and nonverbal interaction" (p. 169). Examples: drama, square dancing, and singing groups.
8. Intergroup: "Action of a competitive nature between two or more intragroups" (p. 170). Examples: team competitions.

Note: These patterns of interaction are important information to monitor and document. They can be instrumental in assessment and goal setting.

COMMUNICATION WITH RESIDENTS IN LEISURE EMPOWERMENT

The therapeutic recreation specialist should monitor all residents during the leisure empowerment session. If the session takes place in a group, the specialist should try to spend some time with each resident. Axline (1969) outlines eight basic principles to follow in the empowerment session.

1. The therapist must develop a warm friendly relationship with the...[resident], in which good rapport is established as soon as possible.
2. The therapist accepts the...[resident] exactly as he [she] is.
3. The therapist establishes a feeling of permissiveness in the relationship so that the... [resident] feels free to express his [her] feelings completely.
4. The therapist is alert to recognize the feelings the...[resident] is expressing and reflects those feelings back to him [her] in such a manner that he [she] gains insight into his [her] behavior.
5. The therapist maintains a deep respect for the...[resident's] ability to solve his [her] own problems if given an opportunity to do so. The responsibility to institute change is the...[resident's].
6. The therapist does not attempt to direct the...[resident's] actions or conversation in any manner. The...[resident] leads the way; the therapist follows.
7. The therapist does not attempt to hurry the therapy along. It is a gradual process and is recognized as such by the therapist.
8. The therapist establishes only those limitations that are necessary to anchor the therapy to the world of reality and to make the resident aware of his [her] responsibility in the relationship.

Leisure empowerment is centered in the present. The specialist focuses on present actions and feelings. These are paraphrased or echoed back to the client. For instance, a resident is interacting with the Bandu game, building odd shaped wooden pieces into a tower. Then she reaches out and smashes it down. The interaction might go something like this:

Therapist: "You smashed the tower down." (Nonjudgmentally)
Resident: "Yes, I did. It was a stupid tower."
Therapist: "You think the tower is stupid." (Matter-of-factly, not judgmentally.)
Resident: "It's stupid and I hate it."
Therapist: "You think the tower is stupid and you hate it." (Note that the therapist does *not* ask why.)
Resident: "Yeah, it reminds me of my house—knocked it down."
Therapist: "The tower reminds you of your house because it got knocked down, and you hate that."
Resident: "Yeah. (Angrily) After I moved here, to this place, my son sold the house to a developer, and he knocked it down and put in a big mall with lots of stores."
Therapist: "You feel angry that your son sold your house to a developer who knocked it down to build a mall."
Resident: "Yeah, there were lots of memories in that house, and now it's all gone."
Therapist: "There were memories in the house, and now the house is gone, and the memories are gone, too." (Note that the therapist does *not* remind the resident that she will always have the memories.)

Resident: "Well, no, the memories aren't gone, but the house is."
Therapist: "The house is gone, but you still have the memories."
Resident: "Yeah, (sadly) I do have the memories, but I'll never be able to go back there, to the house."
Therapist: "You are sad that you will never be able to go back to your house."
Resident: (Cries.) "My husband and I built that house. I was sad when he died, but at least I had the house and the memories. Now they're both gone."
Therapist: "You are sad that the house that you and your husband built together is gone. It reminds you of him."
Resident: "Yes, and now I have nothing."
Therapist: "You feel like you have nothing left."
Resident: "I'm all alone. My son is too busy to visit, and I've got nobody else."
Therapist: "You feel all alone because your son doesn't have time to visit, and there is nobody else who would visit you." (Note that the therapist does *not* say that the resident has the staff, etc., or others. The feelings are simply accepted as valid.)
Resident: "Well, there's my sister, but she's in the nursing home down the line, and she can't get out to visit."
Therapist: "You have a sister but she can't visit you because she's in a nursing home."
Resident: "We used to talk on the phone almost every day. Then we both got sick, her first, and now I haven't heard from her in, oh, quite awhile, now."
Therapist: "You used to talk to your sister every day, but haven't talked to her lately." (Note that the therapist does *not* jump in to provide suggestions or solutions, but allows the resident to process and solve at her own pace.)
Resident: "Yeah, I wonder how she is doing. Maybe I could call her or something."
Therapist: "You are wondering if you could call your sister in the nursing home."
Resident: "Yeah, I'd like to call her and see how she is. Say hello, you know, and talk about things we used to do."
Therapist: "You would like to call your sister and talk with her."
Resident: "Yes, I would really like to do that, but I don't know how I would go about it."
Therapist: "You would like to call your sister, but you don't know how to get in touch with her."
Resident: "Yeah, I don't have a phone number for her—she doesn't have her own phone, you know. I would have to find out a number for the place and see where I could call her."
Therapist: "You want to find a phone number where you can reach your sister." (Note that the therapist does *not* offer to get the number for the resident. It would be appropriate, however, to consent to help *if* the resident asked for it.)
Resident: "Yeah, I know the name of the nursing home, but I don't have a number. I guess I could call the operator or find a phone book and look it up there. There's a phone book by the pay phone on my floor."
Therapist: "You want to look up the phone number for your sister's nursing home in the phone book."
Resident: "Yes, I'm going to do it as soon as I get back to my room."

Several important things about nondirective leisure empowerment can be learned from this example. First, the specialist clarifies and reflects back information and feelings. When the resident hears them being mirrored back to her, she checks them for accuracy, and this helps her clarify not only how she is feeling, but the accuracy of information as well. Second, this technique helps the resident feel that the specialist understands her. Third, this type of communication allows the resident to solve her own problem. The feedback helped her to clarify her feelings of loneliness, and helped her to come up with her own solution. The important lesson to be learned here is that the specialist did not jump in and solve the problem for her. Consider a different scenario where the therapist does jump in ahead of the resident and suggests she call her son or sister, and then offers to find the number, take her to a phone, and place the call for her. Chances are, the resident will refuse claiming it is too much trouble or some similar argument. By allowing the resident to direct the conversation and the agenda, the resident does not fall into a pattern of learned helplessness, but is empowered by her ability to think and function independently, despite her health status or environmental constraints.

By using this nondirective technique of clarifying and reflecting feelings and information, the therapist can empower residents to maintain their sense of self-determination. It is quicker to jump in and offer solutions to the resident, but what a better outcome when patience and empathy prevail! The resident feels understood by the therapist, has solved her own problem, and is motivated to carry through on it on her own. This can only happen if the therapist practices this technique of reflection. It is difficult at first, but with practice it is empowering.

Documentation of Leisure Empowerment

Observations that are important to document in leisure empowerment include choices made by the resident, activity preferences, and social interaction patterns. Significant developments in conversations, such as break through revelations that come to the resident's awareness during the session. Note any significant emotions displayed as well as any physical difficulties experienced. Always document progress toward established goals. It is preferable that a progress note be made following each session. Always document significant progress or changes in attitudes or abilities.

Axline's nondirective play therapy techniques can be adapted for use with older adults residing in the nursing home. This technique is called leisure empowerment, and is consistent with current nursing home guidelines for enhancing self-determination. The nondirective person-centered approach fosters the condition necessary to leisure, perceived freedom. These concepts coordinate well with each other and can provide a leisure empowerment experience for the nursing home resident.

Chapter Eight

Functioning, Themes, and the MDS: Building Blocks for Interventions

As an overview to this section on interventions, functioning, the use of themes, and the Minimum Data Set (MDS) as a basic screening tool will be discussed. A resident's functioning level is an important consideration for the recreation therapist. Themes can be used as a framework to carry out any intervention. The theme concept can provide meaning, excitement, and sense of adventure to the interventions. The MDS is used to gather information and trigger problem areas. It can also serve to guide the recreation therapist in the provision of sensitive interventions.

Interventions as Related to Functioning

All functioning, from being able to feed oneself to interacting socially with others has multiple determinants (Kemp & Mitchell, 1992). The residents' functioning level is important to consider when planning and implementing programs. A resident needs to have a certain level of physical health to complete an activity, or she will not benefit. If a resident does not feel psychologically safe in a program, she probably will not attend or may simply withdraw. If the environment is not properly structured, the resident may not be able to concentrate on the tasks at hand. The relationship among the components of functioning is represented in Figure 8.1.

Figure 8.1 Functioning Components

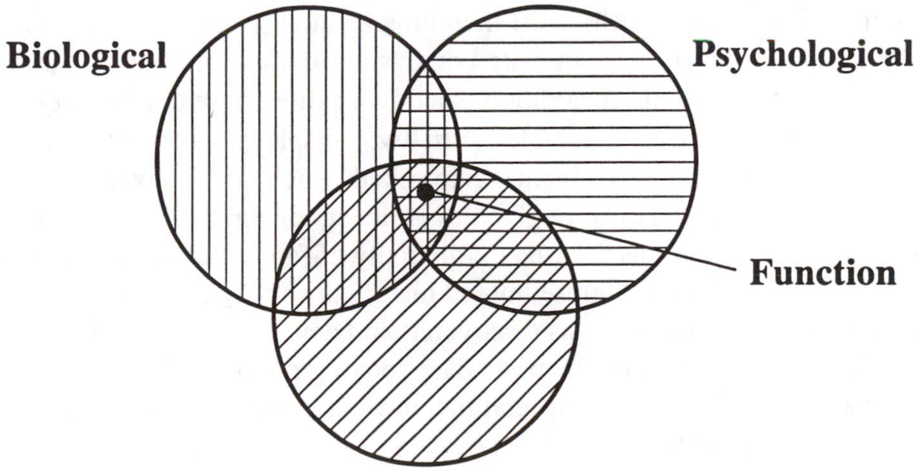

Adapted from Kemp & Mitchell (1992)

Functioning, then, is a product of three distinct areas: biological, psychological and environmental. No aspect of how a resident functions during programs is attributable to only one component however. The three areas overlap and interact with each other. The biological factors that can influence a resident's performance in a program include the presence or absence of illness, strength, flexibility, and the ability to move. Psychological factors include the resident's cognitive ability, motivation and psychosocial skills. Environmental factors such as the amount of light, number of others in the area, excessive noise or clutter, can facilitate or impede performance, especially if the resident is cognitively impaired or physically frail.

The interventions in this section will overlap into all three areas. Specific therapeutic goals and objectives may be different for each resident in the same program. For example, a gardening program may provide the way to work on socialization with one resident. For another resident in the same program, the goal may be to improve strength. The therapist must individually tailor the goals to the residents involved while providing the appropriate activities to achieve them.

Using Themes to Provide Residents with a Purpose

Many just think of aging as a time when one's usefulness declines and one's time is limited. A major intrapersonal constraint to leisure may occur in this situation because the individual does not value leisure activities in general. Activity for activity's sake may not be an option for these residents. To facilitate leisure for the resident who is cognitively impaired or feels useless the therapist may choose to use *themes* in planning and providing interventions.

Each theme may last from a day to a month in length, and all activities focus on the theme selected. Residents in the programs help prepare for the particular event, are encouraged to invite family and friends, and often become personally invested in the event. Creativity and modification of past programming themes is important to entice involvement.

For example, during the week surrounding Columbus Day the theme of "Discover Yourself" was selected by therapy staff and residents. A simple trip to the hairdresser became part of the fun during this theme. The resident was photographed with her regular look before getting a new hairstyle. After the beauty shop visit the resident was asked to select her favorite outfit, and assisted in dressing. The recreation therapist then took an after photograph of the resident with her new look. Before and after shots were mounted on custom-crafted cardboard frames that the resident designed during art group. In addition, shadow profiles were done on selected residents and their family members that were available. A hallway display of the shadow profiles was arranged for the week. Visitors and residents were asked which profiles went together, and answers were collected for fun. Prizes were given to entice involvement in self-awareness. During reminiscence groups the discussions focused on diversity of family histories and where individuals originated. A local speaker from the museum and historical society came to display local artifacts and show slides of how the local area was discovered and developed. A special luncheon was held with a meal of selected favorites from the past. The cooking group made the desserts that were most popular 50 years ago. During this special theme week residents reinvested in their heritage, their looks, and their self-esteem.

Many themes can be used in programming. The easiest ones involve the holidays. Remember, however, the major holidays can bring with them sadness and resentment. The recreation therapist must be ready to assist residents with the grief and other feelings that most likely will surface.

Some of the themes that can be used for programming are listed in Figure 8.2.

Figure 8.2 Programming Themes

-Winter Wonders
-Holidays Around the World
-Chinese New Year
-Winter, Spring, Summer, Fall Solar Celebrations
-Mardi Gras Days
-Luck of the Irish or Leaping Leprechauns
-Earth Day Celebrations
-May Day Around the World
-Maple Syrup Festival
-Declare Your Independence
-Harvest the Community Garden
-State Fair Days
-Going Seaside
-Back to Nature
-Living the Farm Life
-Swedish Mid-Winter Festival
-Indian Summer
-All Hallow's Eve
-Explore the Exotic
-Voting and Claiming your Rights
-The Old Country
-Thanksgiving Turkey Shoot
-Arts Fest
-Grass Roots Festival
-Home Comforts
-Planes, Trains, and Automobiles
-Nordic Life
-The Age of Rediscovery
-Walking Away a Winner
-Where Your Heart Is (Valentine's Day) or Looking for Love
-Choice Adventures
-Filling the Nostalgia Gap

The MDS

The MDS is a screening tool used in all nursing homes to point out residents' problem areas and to give healthcare professionals direction. Often the activities department focuses in on one or two sections of the MDS, such as "Activities" and "Psychosocial." There are, however, several appropriate sections of the MDS that are useful indicators for therapeutic recreation specialists.

Use the MDS Version 2.0 as a guide to the sections that follow. A copy of the MDS can be found in Appendix F.

Chapter Nine

The MDS and Cognitive and Sensory Changes: Issues and Interventions

The next four chapters will follow the MDS section by section and discuss issues and interventions that may be relevant to recreation therapy. It is assumed that the recreation therapist will work as a member of an interdisciplinary team and contribute to all areas of resident care.

Section AC. Customary Routine

On the face sheet of the MDS a section entitled *Customary Routine* is an important place to start in planning therapeutic interventions. Note the resident's cycle of daily activities, eating patterns, ADL patterns, and involvement patterns. If the resident naps every afternoon, do not try to change a routine that he or she may have developed over the past 20 years. Instead, schedule programming at a time when the resident is normally awake and active. Perhaps the resident never engaged in group activities, but enjoyed animal companionship. It would be more important to this resident to attend animal assisted therapy sessions than group social clubs or gatherings. This section of the MDS can give the recreation therapist important insight into the residents' habits and motivations. These should be used as the underlying guide for the implementation of the program schedule.

SECTION AC. CUSTOMARY ROUTINE			
1.	CUSTOMARY ROUTINE *(In year prior to DATE OF ENTRY to this nursing home, or year last in community if now being admitted from another nursing home)*	***(Check all that apply. If all information UNKNOWN, check last box only.)***	
		CYCLE OF DAILY EVENTS	
		Stays up late at night (e.g., after 9 pm)	a.
		Naps regularly during day (at least 1 hour)	b.
		Goes out 1+ days a week	c.
		Stays busy with hobbies, reading, or fixed daily routine	d.
		Spends most of time alone or watching TV	e.
		Moves independently indoors (with appliances, if used)	f.
		Use of tobacco products at least daily	g.
		NONE OF ABOVE	h.
		EATING PATTERNS	
		Distinct food preferences	i.
		Eats between meals all or most days	j.
		Use of alcoholic beverage(s) at least weekly	k.
		NONE OF ABOVE	l.
		ADL PATTERNS	
		In bedclothes much of day	m.
		Wakens to toilet all or most nights	n.
		Has irregular bowel movement pattern	o.
		Showers for bathing	p.
		Bathing in PM	q.
		NONE OF ABOVE	r.
		INVOLVEMENT PATTERNS	
		Daily contact with relatives/close friends	s.
		Usually attends church, temple, synagogue (etc.)	t.
		Finds strength in faith	u.
		Daily animal companion/presence	v.
		Involved in group activities	w.
		NONE OF ABOVE	x.
		UNKNOWN — Resident/family unable to provide information	y.

END

Section A. Identification and Background Information

The information in this section gives the recreation therapist a foundation of information about the resident. The therapist should note the reason for the assessment or reassessment, length of stay in the facility, marital status, and advanced directives. It is particularly important to be cognizant of the advanced directive information during off campus outings. All of these areas, however, can influence the residents' overall functioning in recreation therapy.

SECTION A. IDENTIFICATION AND BACKGROUND INFORMATION

1.	RESIDENT NAME	a. (First) b. (Middle Initial) c. (Last) d. (Jr./Sr.)
2.	ROOM NUMBER	
3.	ASSESS-MENT REFERENCE DATE	a. *Last day of MDS observation period* Month – Day – Year b. Original (0) or corrected copy of form (enter number of correction)
4a.	DATE OF REENTRY	Date of reentry from most recent temporary discharge to a hospital in last 90 days (or since last assessment or admission if less than 90 days) Month – Day – Year
5.	MARITAL STATUS	1. Never married 3. Widowed 5. Divorced 2. Married 4. Separated
6.	MEDICAL RECORD NO.	
7.	CURRENT PAYMENT SOURCES FOR N.H. STAY	*(Billing Office to indicate; check all that apply in last 30 days)* Medicaid per diem a. Medicare per diem b. Medicare ancillary part A c. Medicare ancillary part B d. CHAMPUS per diem e. VA per diem f. Self or family pays for full per diem g. Medicaid resident liability or Medicare co-payment h. Private insurance per diem (including co-payment) i. Other per diem j.
8.	REASONS FOR ASSESS-MENT *[Note—If this is a discharge or reentry assessment, only a limited subset of MDS items need be completed]*	a. Primary reason for assessment 1. Admission assessment (required by day 14) 2. Annual assessment 3. Significant change in status assessment 4. Significant correction of prior assessment 5. Quarterly review assessment 6. Discharged—return not anticipated 7. Discharged—return anticipated 8. Discharged prior to completing initial assessment 9. Reentry 0. *NONE OF ABOVE* b. ***Special codes for use with supplemental assessment types in Case Mix demonstration states or other states where required*** 1. 5 day assessment 2. 30 day assessment 3. 60 day assessment 4. Quarterly assessment using full MDS form 5. Readmission/return assessment 6. Other state required assessment
9.	RESPONSI-BILITY/ LEGAL GUARDIAN	*(Check all that apply)* Legal guardian a. Other legal oversight b. Durable power of attorney/health care c. Durable power of attorney/financial d. Family member responsible e. Patient responsible for self f. *NONE OF ABOVE* g.
10.	ADVANCED DIRECTIVES	*(For those items with supporting documentation in the medical record, check all that apply)* Living will a. Do not resuscitate b. Do not hospitalize c. Organ donation d. Autopsy request e. Feeding restrictions f. Medication restrictions g. Other treatment restrictions h. *NONE OF ABOVE* i.

Section B. Cognitive Patterns

Differential Diagnoses

To understand and provide proper care and treatment it is important that an accurate diagnosis of cognitive and mental health be made. The recreation therapist should be aware of the diagnosis, and plan interventions accordingly. Unfortunately, many nursing home residents are not thoroughly diagnosed in these areas.

It is often difficult to determine if the resident has depression, dementia, or a delirium simply from a therapeutic interaction. A careful history of the course of the disease can give some indication of the diagnosis. For example, if the onset was insidious and the course was of gradual decline Senile Dementia of the Alzheimer's Type (SDAT) is most likely the diagnosis. If the onset was affiliated with a cerebral vascular condition, and the course of the deterioration was stepwise the diagnosis is most likely multi-infarct dementia. Depression is distinguished by "sustained and pervasive disturbances in mood in the presence of clear consciousness" (Birren, Sloane, & Cohen, 1992, p. 633). Delirium is a syndrome of diverse organic causes. The clinical features develop over a short period of time and fluctuate over the period of the day. Depression and delirium can be superimposed on a dementia in some residents.

SECTION B. COGNITIVE PATTERNS			
1.	COMATOSE	*(Persistent vegetative state/no discernible consciousness)* 0. No 1. Yes ***(If yes, skip to Section G)***	
2.	MEMORY	*(Recall of what was learned or known)* a. Short-term memory OK—seems/appears to recall after 5 minutes 0. Memory OK 1. Memory problem **2**	
		b. Long-term memory OK—seems/appears to recall long past 0. Memory OK 1. Memory problem **2**	
3.	MEMORY/ RECALL ABILITY	***(Check all that resident was normally able to recall during last 7 days)*** Current season a. Location of own room b. Staff names/faces c. That he/she is in a nursing home d. *NONE OF ABOVE* are recalled e.	
4.	COGNITIVE SKILLS FOR DAILY DECISION-MAKING	*(Made decisions regarding tasks of daily life)* 0. *INDEPENDENT*—decisions consistent/reasonable 1. *MODIFIED INDEPENDENCE*—some difficulty in new situations only **2** 2. *MODERATELY IMPAIRED*—decisions poor; cues/supervision required **2** 3. *SEVERELY IMPAIRED*—never/rarely made decisions **2, 5B**	
5.	INDICATORS OF DELIRIUM—PERIODIC DISORDERED THINKING/ AWARENESS	*(Code for behavior in the last 7 days.)* [***Note: Accurate assessment requires conversations with staff and family who have direct knowledge of resident's behavior over this time.***] 0. Behavior not present 1. Behavior present, not of recent onset 2. Behavior present, over last 7 days appears different from resident's usual functioning (e.g., new onset or worsening)	
		a. EASILY DISTRACTED—(e.g., difficulty paying attention; gets sidetracked) **1, 17***	
		b. PERIODS OF ALTERED PERCEPTION OR AWARENESS OF SURROUNDINGS—(e.g., moves lips or talks to someone not present; believes he/she is somewhere else; confuses night and day) **1, 17***	
		c. EPISODES OF DISORGANIZED SPEECH—(e.g., speech is incoherent, nonsensical, irrelevant, or rambling from subject to subject; loses train of thought) **1, 17***	
		d. PERIODS OF RESTLESSNESS—(e.g., fidgeting or picking at skin, clothing, napkins, etc.; frequent position changes; repetitive physical movements or calling out) **1, 17***	
		e. PERIODS OF LETHARGY—(e.g., sluggishness; staring into space; difficult to arouse; little body movement) **1, 17***	
		f. MENTAL FUNCTION VARIES OVER THE COURSE OF THE DAY—(e.g., sometimes better, sometimes worse; behaviors sometimes present, sometimes not) **1, 17***	
6.	CHANGE IN COGNITIVE STATUS	Resident's cognitive status, skills, or abilities have changed as compared to status of 90 days ago (or since assessment if less than 90 days) 0. No change 1. Improved 2. Deteriorated **1, 17***	

Reprinted with permission of Briggs Health Care Products, Des Moines, Iowa 50306 • (800) 247-2343

DEMENTIA—What is it?

Dementia is a syndrome, or an umbrella term, that includes a variety of diagnoses in which a primary symptom is memory loss. The most prevalent type of dementia in the nursing home is Alzheimer's disease. Over 50 percent of the dementia cases that occur are of the Alzheimer's type. The next most prevalent form of dementia is the multi-infarct type. Both of these types of dementia are irreversible and cause changes in cognitive and psychosocial functioning. In Alzheimer's disease the progression is gradual and steady. However, in multi-infarct dementia, the progression of the disease plateaus for a period of time, or is step-wise. Some residents may have both types of dementia in a combined form. There are many other causes of dementia, some of which are reversible.

These diseases are not easy to diagnose, and are seldom considered important once the resident is in a long-term care facility. Individuals with Alzheimer's disease or multi-infarct dementia may also have behavioral or psychiatric symptoms that are disruptive in nature.

Therapeutic Programming Needs

Some nursing homes have specialized units for the care and treatment of people with dementia. Other facilities integrate residents with dementia throughout the living units. For those facilities that have special care units, the Joint Commission on Accreditation of Health Care Organizations (1994) has established standards and survey protocols. Although JCAHO certification is voluntary, these standards should be considered when establishing therapeutic or activities programs on special care units in nursing homes. The following regulations from the JCAHO Standards Guide (1994) are the most pertinent to recreation therapy:

PC.11 states that "the activities program provides services that are suited to patients' needs, abilities, and interests" (p. 99). Activities that are considered therapeutic include those that have obvious purpose and meaning for the resident, offer a reasonable chance for success, reestablish old roles, confirm dignity, and are pleasurable. These activities should not add to anxiety, and should be broken into manageable steps that capitalize on remaining abilities. The activities must be culturally appropriate and voluntary. For example, if you have a large number of European immigrant residents, an adapted cooking program entitled "European Cooking Club" may be a good way to meet the regulation and the needs of the participants. Residents in this group would contribute old country recipes and prepare them for the club. Cooking tasks would be broken down into single steps and typed in large print on index cards. Different countries and homelands would be discussed during the sessions.

PC11.1 states that "activities must be provided in individual and group settings for both ambulatory and nonambulatory residents" (p. 100). This regulation is to ensure that bed-bound and nonambulatory residents receive proper programming, opportunities for socialization, and activities. For example, simply providing individualized sensory stimulation two to three times per week may not meet the needs of room-bound patients. Small sensory integration groups mixing ambulatory and nonambulatory residents would allow for socialization with peers. Residents should be encouraged to visit each other outside of program time. The use of the mobile leisure cart on a daily basis is another good way to keep these residents active and involved.

PC11.2 states that "the activities program provides a variety of activities, both inside and outside the facility" (p. 100). Research shows that there are particular programs that are beneficial to dementia patients. These include sensory motor programs, music therapy, art and reminiscence. If you cannot offer these programs at your own facility they may be available in a nearby location in the community. Activities and education sessions that are available in the community should also be made available to residents.

Surveyors will expect that the criteria used in program planning will include an outcome of reduced agitation. Both therapeutic approach and activities to enhance functioning should be addressed. The following activities are encouraged to enhance functioning: therapeutic exercise, recreation and social activities, literary and educational activities, communal activities, spiritual activities, creative activities, intellectually stimulating activities, and other activities to assist patients in maintaining their life styles.

PC11.4 states that "an activities schedule is posted and/or published and is available to all patients, staff, and visitors" (p. 102). It is important to assist families with activities during visits, especially if the resident has difficulty communicating. By including visitors into the programs everyone will have a more positive experience. Programs that have proven success in this area include: family teas, picnics or luncheons; talent shows; evening walking programs, and music-centered activities.

PC11.5 holds that "patients are encouraged to go shopping and participate in community, social, and recreational activities independently, as appropriate" (p. 102). The recreation therapy department should develop policies and procedures to determine which residents are appropriate for community outings. Residents should then be encouraged to pursue these activities. For example, taking a small walking group to a local store is therapeutic and meaningful. Residents should be encouraged to manage small amounts of money and to purchase things they need.

PC11.6 contends that a "variety of supplies and equipment is available to satisfy patients' activity needs and interests" (p. 102-103). Supplies and equipment must be safe for dementia residents and should be age-appropriate. Both inside and outside areas should be available to residents for leisure activities. The wanderers' lounge is a perfect way to provide the supplies and equipment for recreation. Small niches filled with supplies should be conveniently located around the unit for those residents who do not like the larger lounge area or who cannot get there due to mobility losses.

PC11.7 maintains that "patient care policies and procedures serve as a guide to patient activities" (p. 103). A nursing home's policy and procedure manual, quality assurance documents, and care plans should address this area and should guide program development.

Clinical Issues

Because of the functional changes and the behavioral problems associated with cognitive impairment, the older adult with dementia is often unable to benefit from traditional long-term care activities programs. These individuals may become confused and agitated when placed in large group (over five) activities or during transport to programs. The individual with dementia needs step by step directions and just the right amount of stimulation. Residents with dementia are at high risk for potential disuse syndrome, falls, and sensory deprivation. Residents with these diagnoses require specialized programming based on their needs, past interests, and current functioning levels.

Neurologists have shown through experiments that older adults with Alzheimer's-type dementia cannot learn verbal information, rules, or new faces (Eslinger & Damasio, 1986). However, research in therapeutic recreation has lead to some other important findings. For instance, therapeutic programming should be sensorimotor in content (Buettner, 1994). Individuals with chronic dementia can learn motor skills, and improve in the areas of strength, flexibility, and mobility. By using special tips and techniques in providing activities, residents with dementia can experience meaningful leisure. Programmers should use the following information in planning therapeutic activities:

1. *Improve communication.*

   Therapists must focus on the resident and practice active listening skills: eliminate distractions in the environment like a TV or radio in the background before attempting communication, treat each resident as an individual, do not speak to a group, but to each person in the group, do not interrupt the resident who is trying to make a point, no matter how confused it may seem, get in front of the person and at eye level when interacting with him or her. Remember body language can convey tension and impatience to the resident. Use a relaxed expression and simplified visual and verbal cues to help.
2. *Supervise the activity. Don't take it over.*

   Recreation therapists should remember it is the process of active involvement that is important to the resident, not the finished product. The therapist must structure the task so that it is challenging, not frustrating. The resident may need a step-by-step break down of tasks. Written instructions with one step on each page often helps if the resident is able to read.
3. *Normalize the activity schedule.*

   The schedule of activities should fit the normal daily routine. For example, an older adult in the community may enjoy an early morning or evening walk outdoors. A therapeutic walking program may be offered while residents are waiting for breakfast or just after dinner. Along with this idea the therapist should normalize both what she wears, and what the resident wears. The resident might get confused if the therapist comes to the walking group in high heels and a business dress. She also might not realize the aim of the program if she is wearing slippers instead of walking shoes. Post the schedule on the unit, in the resident's room, and give reminder cards to residents who may need them.
4. *Use the rule of inclusion, **not exclusion.***

   Residents with dementia can become agitated if the activity and the environment are not structured to match his or her level of functioning. If there is too much noise or not enough one-to-one communication in the program the resident may become agitated. If the resident is not allowed free movement and an opportunity for physical activity, agitation may result.

   Instead of excluding the resident from recreation programs because of these behaviors, the therapist must adjust the program to meet the resident's needs.
5. *Be prepared to offer a diversion.*

   If a resident becomes bored or agitated in a therapeutic recreation program, attempt to divert his or her attention with a new task. The recreation therapist should make herself a half apron filled with diversional objects in every pocket. For example, during an exercise routine Mr. B. stops working on the tasks provided and becomes verbally abusive. The therapist has a pocket-sized photo album to hand Mr. B. On the cover of the album are the words "LOOK INSIDE." Mr. B. becomes interested and enjoys the pictures of children and animals found inside.

Other ideas to offer as diversions include magnets which are artfully decorated with large pieces of leather and a magnetic board, a pocketbook filled with things to rummage through, a pair of colorful socks with objects hidden inside, old jewelry boxes filled with costume jewelry, an old briefcase full of magazines and wallets with items in every pocket.

6. *Base the program tasks on the residents' current functioning levels.*
   If the program tasks are too easy, the resident will complete them without a challenge and become bored. If the tasks are too difficult, the resident will become confused and frustrated.
7. *Although one-to-one programming is ideal, it not usually practical.*
   The therapist should use small groups of three to five individuals providing one-to-one attention for each task within the group for the best effect. Attempts to get the residents to share objects and communicate with each other will enhance the therapeutic effects of the session.
8. *Every recreation program should offer opportunities for movement and stimulation.*
   Merely attending a program is not enough to benefit the residents. Exercise and movement help to relieve emotional and physical stress. Exercise can reduce illness and agitation. Maintaining or improving strength, flexibility, and mobility skills are important goals that can lead to improved self-care. Therapeutic goals to improve on fitness tests are achievable.
9. *Empower residents by providing simplified and structured choices.*
   The recreation therapist who offers two containers of paint and asks, "Which is your favorite color?" or ask, "Would you like to walk outdoors or indoors today?" puts the resident in charge of the situation. The resident should be able to choose where to recreate and for how long.
10. *The best therapeutic programming is interdisciplinary.*

Nursing staff, therapy staff, and others should use a consistent approach and work together so the daily routine makes sense (see Figure 9.1, page 80).

SAMPLE SPECIFIC GOALS RELATING TO COGNITIVE IMPAIRMENTS/RECREATION THERAPY

1. Mrs. A. will demonstrate improved cognitive functioning in recreation therapy programs as evidenced by an increased attention span from 5 to 15 minutes per session within the next 90 days.
2. Mrs. B. will improve independent decision making during recreation therapy as evidenced by making one simple choice during each program during the next 90 days.
3. Mrs. C. will initiate a selected activity in the leisure lounge when provided with three options, one time per week for the next 90 days.
4. Ms. D. will complete three one-step tasks with verbal prompting during each sensory cooking group.
5. Mr. M. will exercise for 10 minutes free of agitation in three geri-exercise sessions per week.

Figure 9.1 Sample Interdisciplinary Schedule

Morning Routine

6:00-8:00	Morning wake-up—Toileting and dressing for breakfast
7:00-8:00	Early Risers Walking Group
8:00-9:00	Dining room—BREAKFAST
9:00-10:00	Finishing Touches Program (e.g., morning care, shaving, cleaning glasses, checking, hearing aids, make-up and jewelry)
10:00-10:30	M–F Exercise for function group
10:30	Nutrition cart
10:40-11:40	M–F Air mat therapy
11:40-12:00	Dining room sensory game/cognitive activity and prepare for lunch
12:00-1:00	LUNCH

Afternoon Routine

1:00-2:00	Rest time in room or leisure lounge
2:00-2:15	Wake-up and toileting
2:15-2:45	Make your own snack program—Blender cooking
3:00-4:00	Therapeutic Recreation
	M: Photography Club
	T: Community Garden Club
	W: Bibliotherapy Program—Poems, reading, writing
	TH: Art Therapy Program
	F: Animal Assisted Therapy or Kids
	SAT: Table games/adapted bingo
	SUN: Family tea and activities
4:00-5:00	Cognitive Therapy: "Price is Right"
5:00	DINNER

Evening Routine

6:00-6:30	Local news and views (Orientation)
6:30	Toileting and wash-up time
	Leisure lounge open
7:00	Small group activities, family visits, visits with kids, animals, walks outside
8:00-9:30	Hydration—Ready for bed—Sleepy-time music

Delirium

The *Handbook of Mental Health and Aging* (Birren, Sloane, & Cohen, 1992) describes delirium as a reversible organic state that if left untreated can result in permanent brain damage. It is a medical condition that a physician or advanced practice nurse needs to be involved in. It differs from dementia in that it has an abrupt onset. An essential feature is a reduced awareness and attentiveness to the environment. The therapist may see transient shifts in attention or a resident who is easily distracted. This type of change should be reported to medical staff right away.

Sensory Changes

One of the jobs of the recreation therapist in nursing home should be to identify the losses that could effect the resident during programming. A major deleterious effect of aging is sensory loss. Sensory losses greatly affect communication which makes even a simple assessment interview very difficult. Identifying sensory loss is also important to prevent the effects of sensory deprivation.

For example, Mrs. M. has stopped attending her favorite activities. She has been spending more and more time in her room. The facility staff could interpret this behavior as depression or apathy. Upon closer investigation, the recreation therapist found that Mrs. M. could no longer read the activity schedule. Understanding the public address announcements has always been a problem for her due to a major hearing loss. In fact, what has happened to Mrs. M. is that she has become more visually impaired. She could neither read when the activities were taking place nor hear the announced programs.

It is easy to understand from this example how some behaviors associated with sensory changes can interpreted as lack of cooperation or lack of motivation. The next section will describe in more detail some of the diseases and aging processes that could effect the individuals you serve.

Section C. Communication/Hearing Patterns

Hearing

Auditory impairments often occur gradually. The resident may be unaware of the extent of the problem, or how much he or she may be missing. Presbycusis is the term used to indicate hearing loss due to the physiological changes of aging. It is characterized by impairment of: 1) perception of high frequency sounds, 2) sound localization, 3) speech discrimination, 4) ability to understand distorted speech, and 5) the ability to recall long sentences.

Intervention Strategies

When working with a client who is hearing impaired the recreation therapist should:

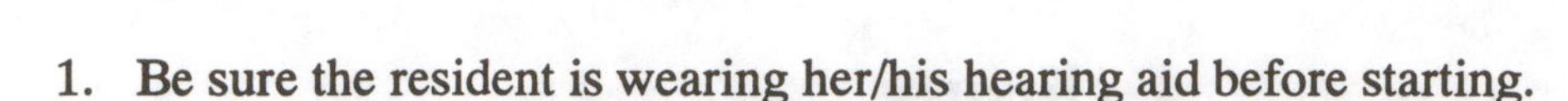

1. Be sure the resident is wearing her/his hearing aid before starting.
2. Ask "Can you hear me?" when beginning to talk to the individual.
3. For clients with high frequency loss, drop the pitch of one's voice.
4. For clients with low frequency loss, raise the pitch of one's voice.
5. Select a quiet working area and turn off the television or radio that may be nearby.
6. Written messages should be used if vision permits.
7. Face the client and talk using a normal voice volume.
8. Use touch if the client is not tactile defensive and trusts his or her therapist.
9. Plan for an extra 10 to 15 minutes per session. Communication takes longer in groups with clients who are hearing impaired.

Suggestions to help promote social activities for clients with hearing impairments include playing cards or table games in small groups; newsletter writing group, cooking, dancing, walking together; using headphones for television or radio groups. A great outing for a small group of older individuals with hearing impairments is a bowling trip. Everyone will be active and involved yet not a lot of verbal communication will be required.

SECTION C. COMMUNICATION/HEARING PATTERNS			
1.	HEARING	*(With hearing appliance, if used)* 0. *HEARS ADEQUATELY*—normal talk, TV, phone 1. *MINIMAL DIFFICULTY* when not in quiet setting 4 2. *HEARS IN SPECIAL SITUATIONS ONLY*—speaker has to adjust tonal quality and speak distinctly 4 3. *HIGHLY IMPAIRED*/absence of useful hearing 4	
2.	COMMUNI-CATION DEVICES/ TECH-NIQUES	***(Check all that apply** during last 7 days)* Hearing aid, present and used Hearing aid, present and not used regularly Other receptive comm. techniques used (e.g., lip reading) *NONE OF ABOVE*	a. b. c. d.
3.	MODES OF EXPRESSION	***(Check all used by** resident to make needs known)* Speech a. Writing messages to express or clarify needs b. American sign language or Braille c. Signs/gestures/sounds d. Communication board e. Other f. *NONE OF ABOVE* g.	
4.	MAKING SELF UNDER-STOOD	*(Expressing information content—however able)* 0. *UNDERSTOOD* 1. *USUALLY UNDERSTOOD*—difficulty finding words or finishing thoughts 4 2. *SOMETIMES UNDERSTOOD*—ability is limited to making concrete requests 4 3. *RARELY/NEVER UNDERSTOOD* 4	
5.	SPEECH CLARITY	*(Code for speech in the **last 7 days**)* 0. *CLEAR SPEECH*—distinct, intelligible words 1. *UNCLEAR SPEECH*—slurred, mumbled words 2. *NO SPEECH*—absence of spoken words	
6.	ABILITY TO UNDER-STAND OTHERS	*(Understanding verbal information content—however able)* 0. *UNDERSTANDS* 1. *USUALLY UNDERSTANDS*—may miss some part/ intent of message 2, 4 2. *SOMETIMES UNDERSTANDS*—responds adequately to simple, direct communication 2, 4 3. *RARELY/NEVER UNDERSTANDS* 2, 4	
7.	CHANGE IN COMMUNI-CATION/ HEARING	Resident's ability to express, understand, or hear information has changed as compared to status of ***90 days ago*** *(or since last assessment if less than 90 days)* 0. No change 1. Improved 2. Deteriorated 17*	

Section D. Vision Patterns

Vision

There are several common diseases of older adults that affect vision. Senile macular degeneration decreases central vision but leaves a ring of peripheral vision. Imagine trying to work on an activity or project on the table in front of you when you only have a ring of outside vision intact. This problem also can affect the resident's ability to eat or to interact with others. Residents with senile macular degeneration function best in a small circle with three to five others. Passing objects or sharing with the person beside her or him is often the most successful arrangement. Using a large upright activity board with bright colors on the outer edges can be developed for the individual with senile macular degeneration.

> For example, if the individual loves to play Monopoly, a wall poster version can be mounted in the activity area. A Velcro strip can be attached to the outer edge of the board, and modified Velcro-backed playing pieces can be used. The cards to draw should be placed on the right or left side on a table. Make a large set of dice to help even more.

Glaucoma is another common disease that affects vision in older adults. It results in the opposite problem. There is a decrease in peripheral vision and sometimes even blindness. It is obvious that a circle activity would be difficult and frustrating for the person with glaucoma unless the therapist provides many adaptations. It would be better in this case to have participants face each other in close proximity. If the lighting is good and the objects used are large and have texture, the individual can be successful.

A good illustration of this is Ms. K. She loves to play dominoes with her grandchildren when they come to visit. Unfortunately her glaucoma has worsened to the point where she could not see the dark small pieces. The recreation therapist recently designed a program with the men's wood crafts group to build large size dominoes for various residents with visual impairments. She knew the color of the large dominoes should be light, and the dots should be textured and raised. Glue and glitter dots work very well. The result was Ms. K. could successfully resume her weekend games with the grandchildren.

Cataracts result in an overall haziness in the visual field. The individual with cataracts has a decreased ability to judge distance and to see in low light levels. High light areas with reflective surfaces are also a problem. For example, Mr. B. had always enjoyed cooking group but when he first entered the bright dining room with the shiny table tops he suddenly became fearful and anxious about attending. The simple adaptation of closing the shades and eliminating confusing reflections solved the problem. Another simple solution, rather than cutting the natural lighting, is to use a cotton table cloth to cut the glare.

In addition to the diseases that cause visual losses, the aging process leads to visual changes. Often an opaque ring develops in the border of the cornea and sclerotic coat. This results in decreases in: 1) general visual acuity; 2) peripheral vision; 3) ability to judge distance; 4) ability to see in bright light when reflections occur; 5) ability to see in low light; 6) ability to discriminate colors, especially blues and greens; and 7) ability to adapt to darkness.

Compensation Strategies

Many of the strategies used by the recreation therapist are based in a common sense approach to residents with visual losses:

1. Avoid startling a resident; when approaching use a verbal greeting.
2. Do not schedule activities in areas with high glare. Be especially mindful of buffed floors and table tops.
3. If programs are provided outdoors, be sure to furnish residents brimmed hats and sunglasses.
4. If natural light comes into the program area, the resident should work with the light to his/her side.
5. When entering a program area always allow time for the resident's eyes to adjust before beginning the activity.
6. Never position the resident so she/he faces the light source.
7. When providing written materials letter height and thickness need to be changed for the resident with visual impairments. Name tags, resident newspapers, signs, schedules should all reflect this.

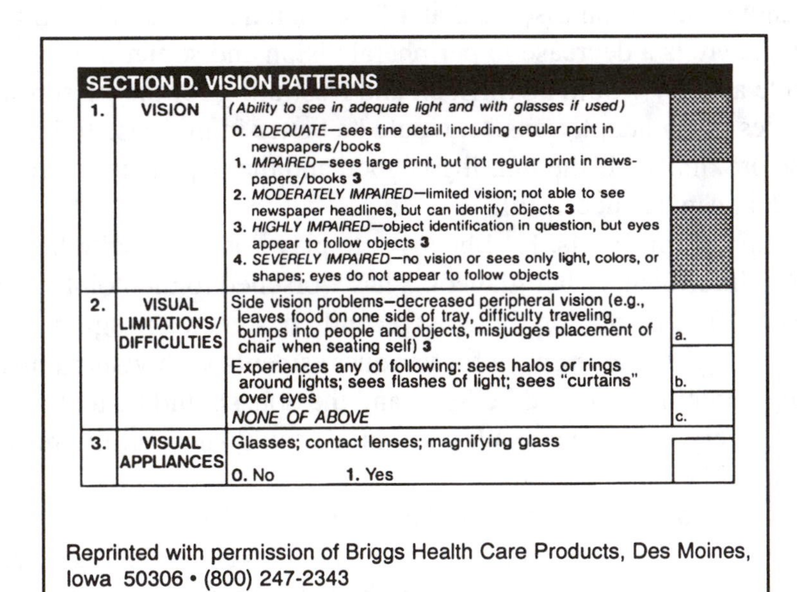

SECTION D. VISION PATTERNS			
1.	VISION	*(Ability to see in adequate light and with glasses if used)* 0. *ADEQUATE*—sees fine detail, including regular print in newspapers/books 1. *IMPAIRED*—sees large print, but not regular print in newspapers/books **3** 2. *MODERATELY IMPAIRED*—limited vision; not able to see newspaper headlines, but can identify objects **3** 3. *HIGHLY IMPAIRED*—object identification in question, but eyes appear to follow objects **3** 4. *SEVERELY IMPAIRED*—no vision or sees only light, colors, or shapes; eyes do not appear to follow objects	
2.	VISUAL LIMITATIONS/ DIFFICULTIES	Side vision problems—decreased peripheral vision (e.g., leaves food on one side of tray, difficulty traveling, bumps into people and objects, misjudges placement of chair when seating self) **3**	a.
		Experiences any of following: sees halos or rings around lights; sees flashes of light; sees "curtains" over eyes	b.
		NONE OF ABOVE	c.
3.	VISUAL APPLIANCES	Glasses; contact lenses; magnifying glass 0. No 1. Yes	

Reprinted with permission of Briggs Health Care Products, Des Moines, Iowa 50306 • (800) 247-2343

Chapter Ten

The MDS and Mood/Behavioral Patterns, Psychosocial Well-Being, and Interventions

Growing older necessitates coping with loss. One's work may appear to be done, friends may die, family members may relocate, one's health may fail, and money may become a problem. Any one of these events can be the stimulus that leads to profound feelings of sadness, and depression may ensue.

Section E. Mood and Behavior Patterns

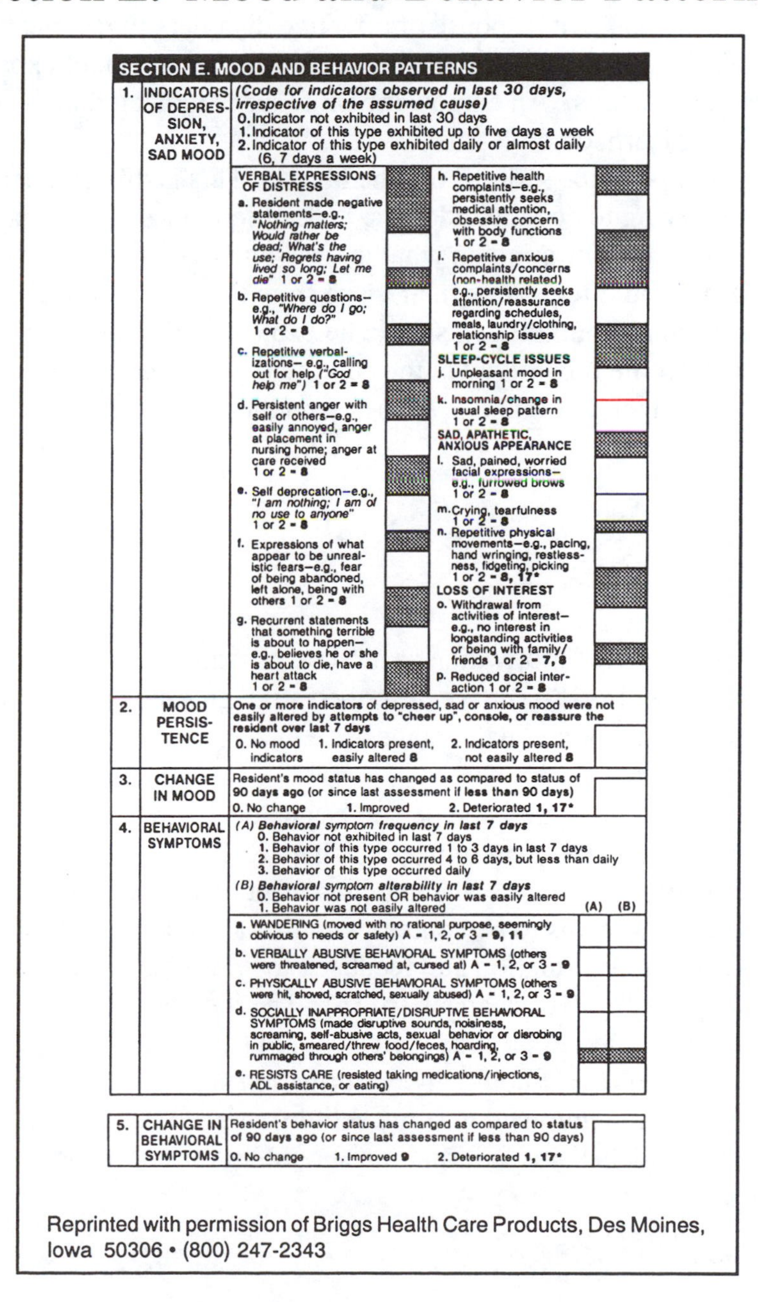

SECTION E. MOOD AND BEHAVIOR PATTERNS

1. INDICATORS OF DEPRESSION, ANXIETY, SAD MOOD

(Code for indicators observed in last 30 days, irrespective of the assumed cause)
0. Indicator not exhibited in last 30 days
1. Indicator of this type exhibited up to five days a week
2. Indicator of this type exhibited daily or almost daily (6, 7 days a week)

VERBAL EXPRESSIONS OF DISTRESS

a. Resident made negative statements—e.g., *"Nothing matters; Would rather be dead; What's the use; Regrets having lived so long; Let me die"* 1 or 2 = 8

b. Repetitive questions—e.g., *"Where do I go; What do I do?"* 1 or 2 = 8

c. Repetitive verbalizations— e.g., calling out for help *("God help me")* 1 or 2 = 8

d. Persistent anger with self or others—e.g., easily annoyed, anger at placement in nursing home; anger at care received 1 or 2 = 8

e. Self deprecation—e.g., *"I am nothing; I am of no use to anyone"* 1 or 2 = 8

f. Expressions of what appear to be unrealistic fears—e.g., fear of being abandoned, left alone, being with others 1 or 2 = 8

g. Recurrent statements that something terrible is about to happen—e.g., believes he or she is about to die, have a heart attack 1 or 2 = 8

h. Repetitive health complaints—e.g., persistently seeks medical attention, obsessive concern with body functions 1 or 2 = 8

i. Repetitive anxious complaints/concerns (non-health related) e.g., persistently seeks attention/reassurance regarding schedules, meals, laundry/clothing, relationship issues 1 or 2 = 8

SLEEP-CYCLE ISSUES

j. Unpleasant mood in morning 1 or 2 = 8

k. Insomnia/change in usual sleep pattern 1 or 2 = 8

SAD, APATHETIC, ANXIOUS APPEARANCE

l. Sad, pained, worried facial expressions—e.g., furrowed brows 1 or 2 = 8

m. Crying, tearfulness 1 or 2 = 8

n. Repetitive physical movements—e.g., pacing, hand wringing, restlessness, fidgeting, picking 1 or 2 = **8, 17***

LOSS OF INTEREST

o. Withdrawal from activities of interest—e.g., no interest in longstanding activities or being with family/friends 1 or 2 = **7, 8**

p. Reduced social interaction 1 or 2 = 8

2. MOOD PERSISTENCE

One or more indicators of depressed, sad or anxious mood were not easily altered by attempts to "cheer up", console, or reassure the resident over last 7 days

0. No mood indicators   1. Indicators present, easily altered **8**   2. Indicators present, not easily altered **8**

3. CHANGE IN MOOD

Resident's mood status has changed as compared to status of 90 days ago (or since last assessment if less than 90 days)

0. No change   1. Improved   2. Deteriorated **1, 17***

4. BEHAVIORAL SYMPTOMS

(A) Behavioral symptom frequency in last 7 days
0. Behavior not exhibited in last 7 days
1. Behavior of this type occurred 1 to 3 days in last 7 days
2. Behavior of this type occurred 4 to 6 days, but less than daily
3. Behavior of this type occurred daily

(B) Behavioral symptom alterability in last 7 days
0. Behavior not present OR behavior was easily altered
1. Behavior was not easily altered

	(A)	(B)
a. WANDERING (moved with no rational purpose, seemingly oblivious to needs or safety) A = 1, 2, or 3 = **9, 11**		
b. VERBALLY ABUSIVE BEHAVIORAL SYMPTOMS (others were threatened, screamed at, cursed at) A = 1, 2, or 3 = **9**		
c. PHYSICALLY ABUSIVE BEHAVIORAL SYMPTOMS (others were hit, shoved, scratched, sexually abused) A = 1, 2, or 3 = **9**		
d. SOCIALLY INAPPROPRIATE/DISRUPTIVE BEHAVIORAL SYMPTOMS (made disruptive sounds, noisiness, screaming, self-abusive acts, sexual behavior or disrobing in public, smeared/threw food/feces, hoarding, rummaged through others' belongings) A = 1, 2, or 3 = **9**		
e. RESISTS CARE (resisted taking medications/injections, ADL assistance, or eating)		

5. CHANGE IN BEHAVIORAL SYMPTOMS

Resident's behavior status has changed as compared to status of 90 days ago (or since last assessment if less than 90 days)

0. No change   1. Improved **9**   2. Deteriorated **1, 17***

Reprinted with permission of Briggs Health Care Products, Des Moines, Iowa 50306 • (800) 247-2343

Depression

Depression is often confused with dementia in older adults. It has many of the same symptoms. Depression is an affective disorder in which causes the resident to be unhappy, pessimistic and self-deprecative. It may be due to an internal conflict and/or unidentifiable event, e.g., loss of something or someone important. A resident with dementia may also have depression.

Depression usually involves reduced motivation, disturbances of appetite, sleep, and sex drives. Residents with depression may display reduced energy, difficulties in thinking, recurrent thoughts of suicide or death. Psychomotor retardation or agitation, depressed mood, and feelings of worthlessness and guilt are other symptoms. Clinical depression generally lasts for weeks or months.

The resident with clinical depression may be on some medication to relieve depressive symptoms. Activities should be structured to increase self-esteem and interaction. Moreover, there is some research showing the positive response of affective disorders to physical activity. Residents may benefit from programs that increase fitness levels through movement experiences. Walking programs have proven efficacious. An empowerment focus is indicated in programming for people with depression or learned helplessness.

Many residents will experience sadness or "the blues." This is different from clinical depression. Residents may be trying to cope with losses, fear, or loneliness. A therapist must "listen well" to these individuals, concentrating on what the person is saying and trying not to make judgments. The resident should receive regular visits from the therapist or from a volunteer. Activity opportunities such as volunteering should be explored with the individual. Volunteering can help the individual become reinvolved in the community and can boost self-esteem. The recreation therapist must remember that this sadness and loneliness may be worse on weekends and holidays.

Motivating Residents

Miller and Rollnick (1991) define motivation as a "state of readiness or eagerness to change" (p. 14). Prochaska and DiClemente (1982) have described strategies for helping people cope with problems in motivation at each of six major stages:

1. *Precontemplation.* In this stage, the person has no desire to change. She or he does not have any awareness of a problem or need to change. For example, a resident may prefer to stay in her room and do nothing. She may just want to sit and stare at the wall, and may even wish to die. She seems to be content with that attitude. Prochaska and DiClemente (1982) suggest giving information and feedback to "raise his or her awareness of the problem and the possibility of change" (p. 16). The therapist should not give suggestions or advice. One might say, to provide feedback, "Mary you look very sad and lonely sitting in here by yourself." Or, one could give information such as "Mary, people who get out of their rooms and become involved in some activity seem to be happier than the residents who don't." The feedback and information should be varied by the therapist reinforcing certain themes.

2. *Contemplation.* In this stage, the resident has some awareness of a problem, and is contemplating change, usually going back and forth between the pros and cons of accepting the problem and changing. For example, a resident may think "I am sad and lonely sitting in my room, but I don't want to go out and be with the other residents. I should be able to stay in my room if I want. If I go out there, I might not like those people. But, if I stay here, I feel bad." One should help tip the balance in favor of change. The therapist should suggest action, encourage the resident to verbalize the debate which is taking place in her mind, and reinforce the positive side.
3. *Determination.* This stage offers "a window of opportunity which opens for a period of time" (p. 17). A resident may decide to do something about a problem, such as trying an activity out of her room. The task for the therapist is to help the resident find an activity that will bring success and enjoyment. If the resident fails to find an appropriate activity, she may revert back to the stage of contemplation.
4. *Action.* At this stage a resident actually takes some action to make a change. The therapist should provide as much assistance as is necessary, especially in planning and implementing the activity, to ensure that the resident's action is successful.
5. *Maintenance.* At this stage, a person who has started a new activity keeps it up. The therapist should identify what the resident needs in order to maintain involvement in an activity. For example, a resident might need a reminder, assistance with transportation, or even help learning new skills.
6. *Relapse.* It is possible for residents to slip into periods of relapse during which some activity is discontinued. One explanation may be that the new activity did not produce desirable outcomes for the person. The therapist should assist the resident by encouraging the resident to find other ways of resolving the problem. The goal is to "help the person avoid discouragement and demoralization, continue contemplating change, renew determination, and resume action and maintenance efforts" (p. 17). For example, a therapist could help a resident choose new activities which would offer greater enjoyment and motivate her to leave her room.

Other Program Ideas

Life review programs are sometimes effective for residents who are mildly depressed. Looking back over past experiences is an essential human need (Butler, 1962). Self-reflection through extensive autobiography work can help residents reconstruct and reevaluate their lives. This program may provide satisfaction and therapeutic benefits for some older persons, but it can also cause renewed despair for others. The therapist must take care as some residents will experience a sense of regret and pain.

Intergenerational programs can help children learn about aging and give residents a place to share life experiences. Involvement with children sometimes brings the most withdrawn and depressed individual into the activity room.

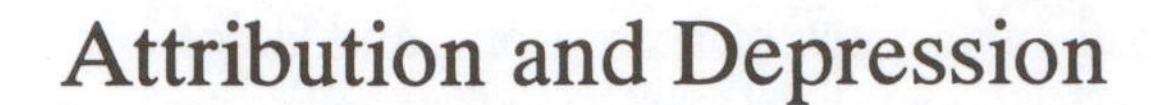

Attribution and Depression

Another important concept in working with older adults with depression is the empowerment process. The therapist's role may mean helping the resident to make positive attributions for her successes or failures. When a person succeeds or fails at an activity, he or she always makes an attribution for it or an explanation as to why. There are four possible types of attributions: ability, effort, task difficulty, and luck. For example a resident may say to herself:

> I lost that game because I'm no good at it (ability),
> I lost that game because I wasn't trying (effort),
> I lost that game because it was to hard (task difficulty), or
> I lost that game because of bad luck (luck).

In general, people who are healthy and not experiencing depression attribute successes to ability or effort. People who have depression generally attribute their successes to luck. It is most helpful when using empowerment to help the resident to attribute successful actions to their ability and effort. This is an internal attribution, that is it happened because of something inside the resident, her ability. It is something she has control over. She can improve her skills and try harder.

If she attributes her success to luck, it is most harmful because it is an external attribution; one which she is unable to control. If a resident fails at an activity, the therapist should encourage increased effort, help her improve skills that will increase her ability, and decrease the task difficulty to insure success.

This attribution theory is also helpful when planning activities for residents. The therapist should choose activities that are based on ability and effort, and activities in which task difficulty is decreased. Programs based on luck do not empower residents, since the outcome can not be controlled; i.e., bingo is an activity based in luck. Success can only be attributed to luck, an external force which the resident has no control over. Instead, the therapist should choose an activity which can be consistent with positive, internally controlled attributes when successful. Some examples include some card games, pool, darts, bowling, and bocce.

Cognitive Impairments, Mood Disorders, Behavior Problems, and Therapeutic Recreation

Some question whether older adults with cognitive impairments, mood disorders, and behavior problems would benefit from therapeutic recreation programs. There are experts in gerontology who argue that participation in activities provides little benefit. Others argue that exposure to activities, at the very least, provides stimulation that helps the older adult maintain skills. These authors believe that therapeutic recreation has the potential to be the treatment of choice for residents with cognitive impairments, mood disorders, and behavior problems or agitation that may result.

Appropriate therapeutic recreation programming for the agitated resident provides several benefits. For example, everyone is concerned about the use of physical and chemical restraints for older adults. Those restraints might be replaced with activities scheduled to take place when agitation is most likely to occur. By doing this, therapeutic programming would help facilities comply with OBRA regulations. Appropriate exercise, stimulation, and activities that promote movement can both improve functioning and reduce agitation. In addition to the physiological benefits, the psychological benefits to the agitated resident are also important. The warm relationship and unique communication that often results from positive leisure experiences can have a calming effect. If the tasks provided during therapeutic recreation are both challenging and interesting, the resident will experience success. This will result in less frustration, isolation, and agitation. Therapeutic recreation programming for those residents who are agitated will also benefit others in the same environment. When one resident is agitated, everyone around him suffers.

What is Agitation?

Disruptive behaviors are any behaviors that disrupt the living or working milieu. Agitated behaviors are more specific, and have been defined as verbal, vocal, or motor patterns that may be due to the confusion or needs of the individual (Cohen-Mansfield & Belig, 1986). Agitation may also be displayed as yelling, making repeated demands or movements that serve no purpose, or destructive behaviors. Aggressive behaviors are even more specific and can be evidenced as verbal or physical behaviors that cause harm to oneself or others. These behaviors have a profound effect on the quality of life for a person with a dementia syndrome. Not only do these behaviors cause acute management problems for caregivers, but also they are often used as a reason to exclude residents from activities and social interactions.

What Causes Agitation?

Little is known about the causes of agitation. Researchers suggest there are certain conditions that may predispose a resident to agitated behavior. These conditions include: 1) lack of exercise, stimulation, or activity, 2) loneliness, 3) depression, 4) needing assistance with activities of daily living, and 5) being restrained. Some gerontologists believe residents are more likely to be agitated at certain times of day. Early morning and early evening hours seem to be especially troublesome periods for cognitively impaired residents. Activities and tasks that are either too easy or too difficult for the resident may lead to frustration and agitation as well.

What Can Be Done?

Therapeutic recreation specialists can be front line players in reducing agitation in long-term care facilities. Instead of using behavior problems as a reason to exclude a resident from programs, the therapist must develop activities to better meet the resident's needs, being aware that there may be a serious biological cause for a resident's agitated behavior. Once medical reasons for agitation have been explored and ruled out, the following treatment approaches are recommended for the therapeutic recreation specialist:

1. Develop a consistent, warm therapeutic relationship and work at improving communication with the resident.
2. Respect the resident's personal space. The agitated individual should not be approached too closely or placed in a crowded activity area.
3. Direct the attention of the agitated individual. One staff member only should calmly speak to the individual and serve as a single source of communication.
4. Give clear, concise directions for even the most simple tasks. The agitated individual may have difficulty with decisions and adaptive responses.
5. Use comfortable positioning, massage, and small group activities that allow for free movement.
6. Promote sufficient rest, sleep, and relaxation. Sensory air mat therapy works well for residents with dementia.
7. Provide consistent, low stimulus physical and social environments.
8. Provide structured programs that assist the individual in retaining a sense of control, responsibility, and usefulness.
9. Structure activity tasks to match the skill levels and tolerance levels of the individuals.
10. Schedule programs to involve the agitated individuals at times when they are anxious or isolated. Therapeutic programs should fit into the schedule of the daily routine to alleviate periods of boredom.
11. Design simple physical activities to provide strength, flexibility, and endurance. These help the individual maintain or improve self-care skills and to feel competent.
12. Minimize environmental changes for programming, and create a controlled environment for walking and wandering. Develop an area which can be used as a leisure lounge.

Section F. Psychosocial Well-Being

The recreation therapist should assist residents in areas involving psychosocial well-being. The sensitive therapist will take great care to promote the residents' involvement in structured leisure time activities and do assist residents in their relationships with others. The recreation therapist can also help residents hold on to or cope with past roles. For example, Ernestine spent most of her adult life working with children as an elementary teacher and tutor. She now feels sad and empty because she no longer has the opportunity to work productively with children. She became so angry about this loss that she had serious conflicts with other residents including her roommate. The recreation therapist developed an afterschool tutoring program for third grade children who were having problems reading in which Ernestine gave reading instruction several days a week. She gained an renewed sense of involvement, and her angry behaviors soon disappeared.

Family Visits, Dementia, and the Recreation Therapist

Unsettled relationships with family members can also be problematic for nursing home residents. Some of the most difficult areas to address involves families of residents' with dementia. Friends and relatives often need support and education before visiting a significant other with dementia so

SECTION F. PSYCHOSOCIAL WELL-BEING			
1.	SENSE OF INITIATIVE/ INVOLVEMENT	At ease interacting with others	a.
		At ease doing planned or structured activities	b.
		At ease doing self-initiated activities	c.
		Establishes own goals 7	d.
		Pursues involvement in life of facility (e.g., makes/keeps friends; involved in group activities; responds positively to new activities; assists at religious services)	e.
		Accepts invitations into most group activities	f.
		NONE OF ABOVE	g.
2.	UNSETTLED RELATIONSHIPS	Covert/open conflict with or repeated criticism of staff 7	a.
		Unhappy with roommate 7	b.
		Unhappy with residents other than roommate 7	c.
		Openly expresses conflict/anger with family/friends 7	d.
		Absence of personal contact with family/friends	e.
		Recent loss of close family member/friend	f.
		Does not adjust easily to change in routines	g.
		NONE OF ABOVE	h.
3.	PAST ROLES	Strong identification with past roles and life status 7	a.
		Expresses sadness/anger/empty feeling over lost roles/status 7	b.
		Resident perceives that daily routine (customary routine, activities) is very different from prior pattern in the community 7	c.
		NONE OF ABOVE	d.

Reprinted with permission of Briggs Health Care Products, Des Moines, Iowa 50306 • (800) 247-2343

that visits do not become a negative experience. The therapeutic recreation specialist can play an important role in promoting positive family visits. Often, when a visitor arrives, the resident is hastily prepared and wheeled off to a visiting area. The older person with dementia is placed in a strange room with one or more uncomfortable visitors who do not know what to do next. With this scenario in mind the following list of recommendations would seem appropriate:

1. Visits should occur in a familiar area with a controlled environment for walking or wandering nearby. For example, a visit could start in the resident's room and finish with a walk outside.
2. A recreation therapist or social worker should assist the visitors by providing suggestions and materials for activities that involve the older person with dementia. When the visit nears completion, the entire group should join a unit activity program. The family can then leave discretely once the resident is involved.
3. Activities should match the individual's interests, allow for repetitive gross motor movements, stimulate sensory systems, allow for a sense of control, and make use of long-term memory. Examples include going for a walk to collect flowers or leaves, petting an animal, playing ball with a child, turning the pages of a family album, folding clothes, shuffling and dealing cards, washing off surfaces, writing/drawing on a chalkboard and erasing it, stirring a bowl of cookie dough, and shaking a batch of popcorn.
4. If the individual becomes agitated, redirect his or her attention. Only one person should speak calmly, at eye level to the person. This sole visitor should serve as a single source of communication. Too many people trying to intervene only makes the situation worse. Simplify and restructure the stimulation the older adult is receiving.

Chapter Eleven

The MDS and Physical Issues and Interventions

Section G. Physical Functioning and Structural Problems

SECTION G. PHYSICAL FUNCTIONING AND STRUCTURAL PROBLEMS

1. (A) ADL SELF-PERFORMANCE—***(Code for resident's PERFORMANCE OVER ALL SHIFTS during last 7 days—Not including setup)***

0. *INDEPENDENT*—No help or oversight—OR—Help/oversight provided only 1 or 2 times during last 7 days
1. *SUPERVISION*—Oversight, encouragement or cueing provided 3 or more times during last 7 days—OR—Supervision (3 or more times) plus physical assistance provided only 1 or 2 times during last 7 days
2. *LIMITED ASSISTANCE*—Resident highly involved in activity; received physical help in guided maneuvering of limbs or other nonweight bearing assistance 3 or more times—OR—More help provided only 1 or 2 times during last 7 days
3. *EXTENSIVE ASSISTANCE*—While resident performed part of activity, over last 7-day period, help of following type(s) provided 3 or more times:
   —Weight-bearing support
   —Full staff performance during part (but not all) of last 7 days
4. *TOTAL DEPENDENCE*—Full staff performance of activity during entire 7 days
8. *ACTIVITY DID NOT OCCUR* during entire 7 days

(B) ADL SUPPORT PROVIDED—***(Code for MOST SUPPORT PROVIDED OVER ALL SHIFTS during last 7 days; code regardless of*** *resident's self-performance classification)*

0. No setup or physical help from staff
1. Setup help only
2. One person physical assist
3. Two+ persons physical assist
8. ADL activity itself did not occur during entire 7 days

			(A) SELF-PERF	(B) SUPPORT
a.	BED MOBILITY	How resident moves to and from lying position, turns side to side, and positions body while in bed A - 1 - **5A**; A - 2, 3, or 4 - **5A, 16**; A - 8 - **16**		
b.	TRANSFER	How resident moves between surfaces—to/from: bed, chair, wheelchair, standing position (EXCLUDE to/from bath/toilet) A - 1, 2, 3, or 4 - **5A**		
c.	WALK IN ROOM	How resident walks between locations in his/her room A - 1, 2, 3, or 4 - **5A**		
d.	WALK IN CORRIDOR	How resident walks in corridor on unit A - 1, 2, 3, or 4 - **5A**		
e.	LOCOMOTION ON UNIT	How resident moves between locations in his/her room and adjacent corridor on same floor. If in wheelchair, self-sufficiency once in chair A - 1, 2, 3, or 4 - **5A**		
f.	LOCOMOTION OFF UNIT	How resident moves to and returns from off unit locations (e.g., areas set aside for dining, activities, or treatments). If facility has only one floor, how resident moves to and from distant areas on the floor. If in wheelchair, self-sufficiency once in chair A - 1, 2, 3, or 4 - **5A**		
g.	DRESSING	How resident puts on, fastens, and takes off all items of street clothing, including donning/removing prosthesis A - 1, 2, 3, or 4 - **5A**		
h.	EATING	How resident eats and drinks (regardless of skill). Includes intake of nourishment by other means (e.g., tube feeding, total parenteral nutrition) A - 1, 2, 3, or 4 - **5A**		
i.	TOILET USE	How resident uses the toilet room (or commode, bedpan, urinal); transfers on/off toilet, cleanses, changes pad, manages ostomy or catheter, adjusts clothes A - 1, 2, 3, or 4 - **5A**		
j.	PERSONAL HYGIENE	How resident maintains personal hygiene, including combing hair, brushing teeth, shaving, applying makeup, washing/drying face, hands, and perineum (EXCLUDE baths and showers) A - 1, 2, 3, or 4 - **5A**		

2.	BATHING	How resident takes full-body bath/shower, sponge bath, and transfers in/out of tub/shower (EXCLUDE washing of back and hair). *Code for most dependent in self-performance and support.* A = 1, 2, 3 or 4 **=5A** (A) BATHING SELF-PERFORMANCE codes appear below. (A) (B) 0. Independent—No help provided 1. Supervision—Oversight help only 2. Physical help limited to transfer only 3. Physical help in part of bathing activity 4. Total dependence 8. Activity itself did not occur during entire 7 days *(Bathing support codes are as defined in **Item 1, code B above**)*
3.	TEST FOR BALANCE (See training manual)	*(Code for ability during test in the **last 7 days**)* 0. Maintained position as required in test 1. Unsteady, but able to rebalance self without physical support 2. Partial physical support during test; or stands (sits) but does not follow directions for test 3. Not able to attempt test without physical help a. Balance while standing b. Balance while sitting—position, trunk control 1, 2, or 3 = **17***
4.	FUNCTIONAL LIMITATION IN RANGE OF MOTION (see training manual)	*(Code for limitations during **last 7 days** that interfered with daily functions or placed resident at risk of injury)* *(A) RANGE OF MOTION*: 0. No limitation; 1. Limitation on one side; 2. Limitation on both sides (B) *VOLUNTARY MOVEMENT*: 0. No loss; 1. Partial loss; 2. Full loss (A) (B) a. Neck b. Arm—Including shoulder or elbow c. Hand—Including wrist or fingers d. Leg—Including hip or knee e. Foot—Including ankle or toes f. Other limitation or loss
5.	MODES OF LOCOMOTION	***(Check all that apply during last 7 days)*** Cane/walker/crutch a. Wheeled self b. Other person wheeled c. Wheelchair primary mode of locomotion d. *NONE OF ABOVE* e.
6.	MODES OF TRANSFER	***(Check all that apply during last 7 days)*** Bedfast all or most of time **16** a. Bed rails used for bed mobility or transfer b. Lifted manually c. Lifted mechanically d. Transfer aid (e.g., slide board, trapeze, cane, walker, brace) e. *NONE OF ABOVE* f.
7.	TASK SEGMENTATION	Some or all of ADL activities were broken into subtasks during **last 7 days** so that resident could perform them 0. No 1. Yes
8.	ADL FUNCTIONAL REHABILITATION POTENTIAL	Resident believes he/she is capable of increased independence in at least some ADLs **5A** a. Direct care staff believe resident is capable of increased independence in at least some ADLs **5A** b. Resident able to perform tasks/activity but is very slow c. Difference in ADL Self-Performance or ADL Support, comparing mornings to evenings d. *NONE OF ABOVE* e.
9.	CHANGE IN ADL FUNCTION	Resident's ADL self-performance status has changed as compared to status of **90 days ago** (or since last assessment if less than 90 days) 0. No change 1. Improved 2. Deteriorated

Reprinted with permission of Briggs Health Care Products, Des Moines, Iowa 50306 • (800) 247-2343

Therapeutic Recreation to Prevent Falls

All healthcare professionals should be aware of the risks associated with falls in the elderly and know how to prevent them. It is especially relevant to recreation therapy because the fear of falls can be a major constraint to leisure. A recreation therapy program to prevent falls deals with both the environment in which the program is conducted and with the resident who attends them.

Who? Any resident who has poor balance, sensory loss, an unsteady gait, or a cognitive impairment is a good candidate for falls-prevention programming. If a resident has two falls in any single month, she should be immediately evaluated for falls-prevention programming.

What? Much of what is done in a falls-prevention program is common sense. It is a program to make all activity areas safe and to strengthen the mobility skills of the resident. Falls-prevention exercise groups, morning or evening walking programs, and activities that promote balance should all be included.

Where? Most residents fall in areas of high traffic. Falls occur most often in the bedroom, followed by the bathroom, lounge and dining room. Program entrance areas are often the scene of falls. How residents arrive and leave the program area should be carefully planned to avoid extra confusion.

When? Each resident is different. The therapist should evaluate falls incident reports for each resident in the program. The time of day the resident fell should be noted on each report and may indicate a pattern. Once a resident is deemed "at risk" for falls-prevention programming, he or she should continue in the program until a change in mobility has been established.

Why? Falls are a leading cause of injury and death in older people. A quarter of a million people suffer hip fractures each year. Many of these falls can be prevented. In addition, falls and fear of falling is a major constraint to leisure for older adults.

Preventing Falls in Residents

The best way for the therapeutic recreation specialist to prevent falls is to know each resident, and be alert for changes (*Focus on Geriatric Care and Rehabilitation,* 1987). Difficulties may become apparent during daily, routine walks with residents. Each client has individual strengths and weaknesses which may change daily, weekly, or less frequently. For example, some clients are independent during the day, but become confused at night and require fall precautions. Others may sleep safely through the night, but tend to fall when they get out of bed. The incident reports will reflect this information.

The therapist should communicate any observations to other staff members. Elderly residents often require a structured daily routine, and it is less confusing if every caregiver follows the same precautions. An interdisciplinary schedule and staff information sharing can prevent many falls.

Residents should be protected from environmental hazards, such as scatter rugs, movable furniture, or other unsafe obstacles in program areas. (This is particularly relevant if a program is in the community.) If a resident becomes incontinent or spits on the floor, the area must be cleaned immediately. Lighting should be adequate without creating glare. Leaving a low light on in the resident's room at night may help to decrease confusion.

If a resident complains of dizziness or weakness, he or she should return to bed with the therapist's assistance and the unit nurse should be notified. A resident who is confused or lashing out should have someone stay with him or her for further evaluation. This reassures and protects the resident.

When a resident falls, there are set procedures to be followed. The resident should not be moved until he or she is checked for serious injury. Hip injuries (and pain) are a common result of falls. If the resident complains of pain anywhere, gentle probing with fingertips should be done to the injured area. Increased pain indicates that the client may have a fracture. A loss of consciousness or increased confusion could indicate a head injury. The resident should be checked for bruising or cuts on the head, arms, legs, and hips while the therapist provides reassurance. The therapist should stay with the resident until he or she can be safely moved. Residents who cannot be moved immediately should be covered with a blanket. Unless there is an environmental danger such as a fire, the resident should not be moved by the therapist without additional assistance by another caregiver (*Focus on Geriatric Care and Rehabilitation,* 1987).

Falls Alert

Research shows that certain diagnostic categories have a greater potential for falls. A therapist should be especially vigilant with residents who have any of the following medical conditions: Parkinson's disease, stroke, dementia (cognitive impairment), extracranial artery disease, cardiac disease, dehydration, occult bleeding, hypotension, or foot problems. Other health-related problems that often result in falls include use of psychotropic medications, incontinence, agitation and attempts to get up or get away, and decreased general mobility and strength. Finally, the research shows specific environmental factors associated with falls: glossy floors, improper footwear, unstable furniture, unlocked bed or wheelchair, inadequate lighting, loose rugs, lack of adapted equipment for bathing/toileting, excessive clutter and confusion in the environment, and negotiating stairs.

These environmental factors need to be addressed in the quality assurance manual for recreation therapy. All recreation therapy program areas should be screened routinely for risk factors.

Risk Factors and Interventions

Those residents considered at *high-risk* for falls are usually over 75 years of age, have multisystem disease, use a wheelchair part of the time, are a new admission, and are taking many medications. They may be confused, impulsive, or have a dementia syndrome. They are weak, move slowly and unsteadily, and usually have a history of falls. These residents need: opportunities to move about; constant supervision when walking, transferring, or in the bathroom; the opportunity to build endurance and strength through sensorimotor activities; a chance to become familiar with the environment and the daily routine; and an environment free of glare, clutter, loose rugs, and unsteady furniture.

Residents considered at *moderate-risk* for falls function fairly well, but have periods of increased risk (e.g., after medical procedures, during activities of daily living, when carrying something, or during nighttime toileting). These residents require: assistance at specific times, communication with staff members about special times extra care is needed, ongoing assessment for changes in risk level, education about use of assistive devices, dangling (i.e., sitting on the edge of the bed for a few moments before getting up), and the chance to build endurance and strength through therapeutic activities.

Low-risk residents may have mild physical impairments, but are alert and oriented. They are aware of their deficit and are able to understand and follow instructions. These clients require orientation to sitting, emphasis on provisions for physical needs and how to ask for help with needs, continued assessment for fall risk, education about dangling and transfer techniques, assistive devices, limits for carrying things, careful observation when medications are changed or if his or her condition worsens, and the chance to build endurance and strength through therapeutic activities.

Sensorimotor Programs

It is easy to see from the descriptions above, all residents need programs that provide an opportunity to build strength and endurance. Regularly scheduled exercise programs which are designed to improve functioning are vital. Simply buying a preplanned chair exercise tape is not sufficient for residents with multiple impairments. Each resident differs in ability. Carefully planned small group exercise should include individual attention to each and every resident. This exercise program can be planned with the residents' favorite musical accompaniment. The therapist should be centrally located to demonstrate each movement and to provide assistance to each resident as needed. The routine should follow these guidelines:

EXERCISE FOR FUNCTION

1. Assess each resident for strength, flexibility, endurance, and ability to follow verbal and demonstrated directions.
2. Use a small group set-up for exercise with the therapist rotating to each resident for each movement. This allows for individualized attention and built in rest periods. Exercise starts at the top of the body and continues on down through the legs and feet (i.e., development approach).
3. Start the exercise program by gaining the residents' alertness levels and attention. Pass an object to smell or touch or something to taste.
4. Use a 5/8" dowel or a towel to promote bilateral movements of the upper extremities. Use movements that are used in dressing (e.g., reaching overhead and toward feet) and eating (e.g., bringing hands bilaterally to face or head).
5. Follow bilateral movements with movements of just one arm, swinging a scarf or an exercise flag. Pass the scarf or flag from one hand to the other during the routine. Finally, pass a plastic milk jug from resident to resident for strengthening and balance. A full gallon jug weighs 8 pounds. Start with two to three inches of colored water and add more as the residents gain strength.
6. Use trunk movements next to promote good sitting balance and the ability to adjust posture independently. A good way to do this is by rocking side-to-side, forward and back, in the chair while using the arms for support to adjust posture.
7. Lower extremities are warmed up with dangling leg movements. Residents should then be assisted to do arm chair push-ups. The therapist must encourage the use of the upper legs in the movement to rise from the seat of the chair. The therapist should guard each resident as she completes these movements to prevent a fall forward.
8. For additional lower extremity exercise use an elastic band with a loop sewn in each end. Loop one end around the instep of the foot and hold the other end. Complete leg lifts with the elastic bands while holding the hand steady. Then hold the foot to the floor and reexercise the arm/hand. Any of the lower extremity exercises can be done with ankle weights for added difficulty.
9. Finish with an active game in which the residents are asked to react to a moving object. A suspended therapy ball that is used for a tethered volleyball game is one example. This activity requires the resident to think and quickly respond. It can be graded by using a slower moving large therapy balloon, a suspended ball, and finally a free-moving ball.

10. Residents should be assisted to walk back to their rooms after a cool drink is shared by the group. Walking or wheeling one's own chair is part of the program and should not be omitted.

OTHER SUGGESTIONS

- Don't let your exercise program stagnate: change music, go outdoors in the summer months, or have the residents make the equipment for the program. Grade the routine so the difficulty levels increase as the residents gain strength and endurance.
- Simple gains in strength and flexibility may not give the therapist an accurate picture of the resident's level of overall functioning. Another good assessment tool is the Timed Manual Performance Test. This test is fun for the resident to complete and only takes about 5 minutes of the therapist's time. The tool can be made at the nursing home for under $50 (see Chapter Two).

EXERCISE EQUIPMENT

- clothes pins and brightly colored plastic streamers to make exercise flags
- 1" wide elastic to make exercise stretch bands
- 1/2 and 1 gallon plastic milk jugs
- 5/8" dowel or towels
- ankle weights or heavy bands (optional)
- therapy balloon or balls

Resident goals related to falls prevention programming:

1. Mrs. A. will participate in morning walking group three times a week for 6 weeks to increase her endurance. Mrs. G. will ambulate 100 yards independently for three sessions before discharge from the falls prevention program.
2. Mrs. B. will exercise for 20 minutes two times a week to increase strength, flexibility, and balance.
3. Mrs. C. will demonstrate increased strength and flexibility as evidenced by monthly testing.
    a. Strength will be increased from 2.5 pounds to 4 pounds on the strength test.
    b. Flexibility will be increased from 7 inches to 10 inches on the Modified Wells Bench Test.
4. Mrs. D. will demonstrate safe ambulation by independently walking to and from all recreation therapy programs during the next 90 days.
5. Mrs. E. will be free from falls as evidenced by monthly incident reports.

Sensory Air Mat Therapy

In talking with residents who are mobility impaired about what he or she would like to do in recreation, a common response is "to get out of this chair." One way to help the resident do this and achieve many other TR goals is to set up a sensory air flow mat program.

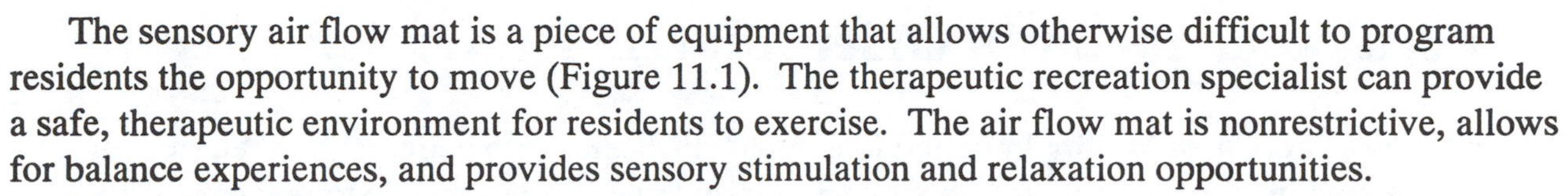

The sensory air flow mat is a piece of equipment that allows otherwise difficult to program residents the opportunity to move (Figure 11.1). The therapeutic recreation specialist can provide a safe, therapeutic environment for residents to exercise. The air flow mat is nonrestrictive, allows for balance experiences, and provides sensory stimulation and relaxation opportunities.

The activities on the air flow mat fall into several specific areas to improve total body movement, reduce agitation or stress levels, and enhance overall functioning. Goals of the program include:

1. Communication links between therapist and resident can be improved.
2. The developmental movements provided in the program can lay the foundation for improving activities of daily living (ADLs).
3. Body awareness skills help the resident understand his/her relative position in space.
4. Improving balance or the ability to maintain one's equilibrium while engaging in various activities like striking a therapy balloon or transferring.
5. Improving vestibular and proprioceptive processing through neurophysiological stimulation.
6. Improving transfer or ambulation skills.
7. Developing a sense of control and confidence in one's self.
8. Reducing stress and levels of agitation.
9. Improving strength, flexibility, and endurance levels.

See Resources, page 141, for purchasing information regarding air flow mats.

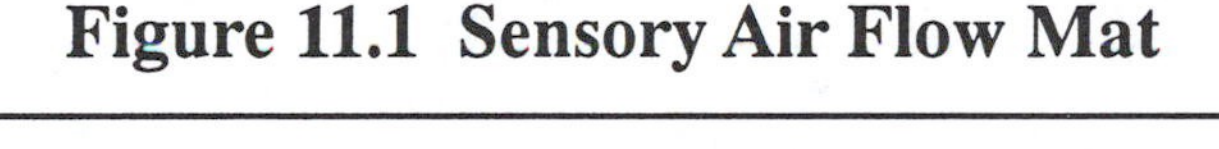

Figure 11.1 Sensory Air Flow Mat

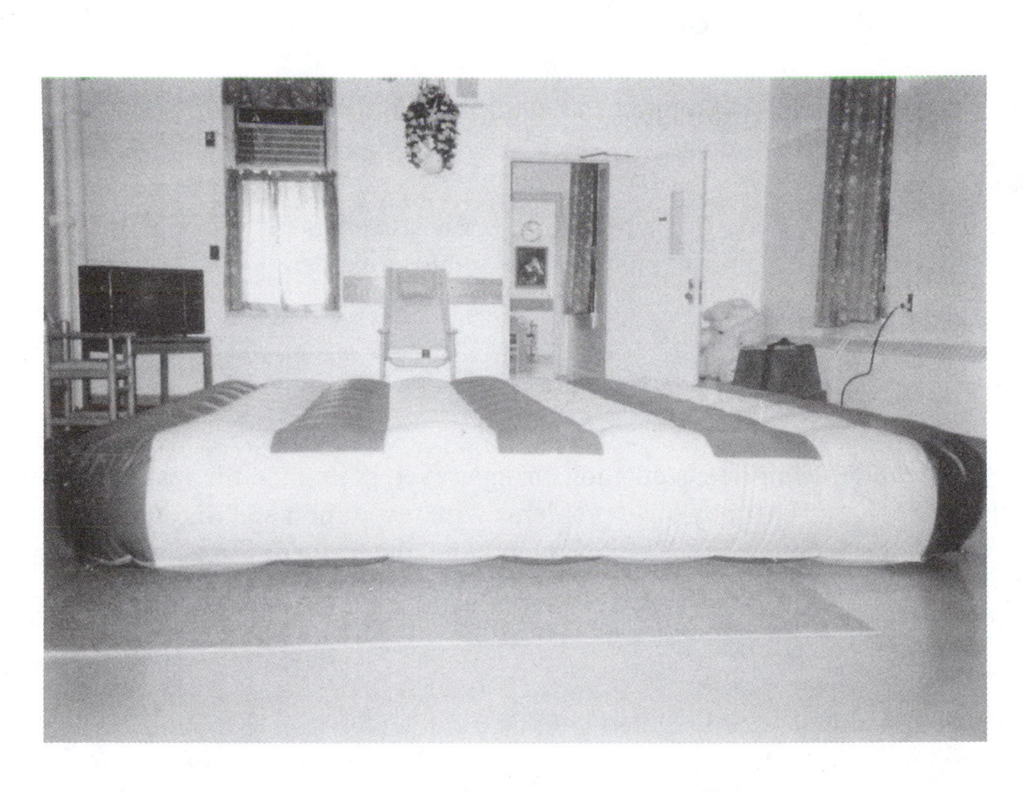

Positioning the Frail Older Adult in Recreation Therapy

The scenario where the mobility impaired individual is wheeled into a recreation therapy program and does not actively participate is common. The individual is often unable to reach or do the things required to take part. She often either falls asleep or becomes frustrated and agitated. Often a simple mistake in thinking is made that "just getting the resident there is enough."

When a recreation therapist brings a resident into her program, the first thing she must do is to create a climate of acceptance and comfort. This has not only a psychological component, but it also has a physiological one. That involves changing the residents' positioning for activity. Help the resident find a comfortable position from which to "recreate." For the resident who ambulates this is not difficult. However, for the resident in a wheelchair or gerichair the task is more challenging.

Tips for Performing a Wheelchair Transfer

- Use brakes during all transfers.
- Tell the resident what is about to be done and how she should help.
- Give support only where needed; let the resident do as much as possible for herself.
- Make the resident aware of her feet before assisting her to stand. Older adults often have poor circulation and kinesthetic sense in lower extremities.
- Remind the resident to lead with her head. She should look to the spot she is going to.

For the Therapist's Safety:

- Keep the back straight and avoid bending forward at the waist.
- Lift using the legs for strength.
- Lift slowly and steadily.
- Keep the resident close to one's body with one's arms bent.
- For a two or three person lift count to three and lift together.

If the Resident is in a Recliner Chair

The resident in a recliner chair needs position changes even more than the residents in wheelchairs or using assistive devices. She may have problems with respiration and digestion because there is no gravity to aid in these functions. If reclined too much the resident is encouraged to rest rather than work on building body control. When a chair is reclined, the visual field is changed and the resident is often looking at the ceiling. The "lying back" position makes normal movements and activity more difficult.

Suggestions

1. Try to keep the resident as upright as possible.
2. The reclining position is acceptable for short periods.
3. For a change in position:
    - Use a pillow under her head and shoulders;
    - Place hips and knees in a flexed and abducted position (bent and separated); and/or
    - Use bean bag chairs which are excellent for small group work. Residents are safe and comfortable.

When working with a resident in bed, try positioning her on her side with a pillow under her head and a pillow between her knees to gain alertness and a position change for activity.

Potential Disuse Syndrome

Potential Disuse Syndrome (PDS) is a state in which an individual is at risk for the complications of prescribed or unavoidable immobilization (Carpenito, 1992). Potential complications include: pressure ulcers, constipation, stasis of pulmonary secretions, thrombus formation, urinary tract infections, decreased strength and endurance, othostatic hypotension, decreased joint range of motion, disorientation, powerlessness, and body image disturbance.

Many of the therapeutic programs provided by recreation therapists in nursing homes can address the complications of PDS. Within the recreation therapy assessment the therapist should identify "at risk" residents. The recreation therapy care plan should then include:

- Programs to promote independence in mobility;
- Activities to increase strength and endurance;
- Opportunities to make simple choices;
- Opportunities to change position frequently;
- Opportunities for appropriate stimulation;
- Opportunities to bear weight;
- Cuing (verbal and physical) for orientation and activities in familiar surroundings; and
- Small group programming with one-to-one attention within each small group.

SAMPLE GOALS

1. Mr. A. will maintain his mental status score throughout his period of prescribed bedrest as evidenced by pretest and posttest Mini Mental State Score.
2. Mr. B. will independently position himself in bed, with cueing from the therapist, before each activity session begins.
3. Mr. C. will make one choice regarding daily activities when provided with two choices each morning.

4. Mr. D. will change positions with the assistance of his therapist every 20 minutes during each 60-minute therapeutic recreation program.
5. Mr. W. will greet two other residents during sensory group programming.
6. Mr. X. will remain free from injuries from falls during the period 4 weeks after his prescribed bedrest terminates.
7. Mr. S. will stand and bear weight to transfer from his wheelchair to a straightback chair in the leisure lounge one time daily.
8. Mr. M. will independently ambulate from his room to recreation therapy programs held on the unit once a day.
9. Mr. N. will make two suggestions for group outings during the summer months in the seasonal recreational planning meeting.

Programming for the Bedridden Resident

A. Mobile leisure carts can be developed with shelves full of equipment, books, magazines, games, headphones and music, craft and sensory items, and more. This cart and a trained volunteer should visit residents who cannot attend other programming on a daily basis.

B. Leisure apron or briefcase can be individually tailored to the needs and interests of residents. Using the persons' lifestyle from the past, make a briefcase or an apron full of activities and objects for stimulation. Include garden gloves, a sponge, music boxes, magazines, koosh balls, jewelry, small photo albums, and an old watch or wallet. Old purses are also excellent. Fill them with safe things to rummage through, and meaningful things from the resident's past. These should be made available to the resident who can not seek out his or her own stimulation and leisure time activities.

C. The sensory motor stimulation center (stim box) was designed to maintain, restore, or develop the basic functions of the upper extremities (see Figure 11.2). It also provides visual, auditory, and tactile, and proprioceptive stimulation. It creates an opportunity to make choices and to understand that one's actions have an effect.

Hand functioning and sensory input are vitally linked. There are many sensory receptors in the hands. Stimulating these receptors helps the resident perform integrated actions. These actions are needed for many recreational pursuits as well as activities of daily living. The basic hand actions that can be developed with this tool include: 1) reach-touch, 2) grasp-push, 3) forearm rotation and carry, and 4) release.

This therapy tool can be built from inexpensive materials found at any electronics store. The stim box supplies numerous sensory receptors with touch, pressure, and position sense. This stimulation tool allows the resident to seek out interesting activities and provides immediate rewards. This tool can be therapist guided or the resident can be encouraged to explore the various objects on her own.

recreation therapist should be aware of these diagnoses, and the appliances and programs
ay be used to treat them. The therapist should be familiar with toileting procedures for the
nts in her program in the event the resident needs to go to the bathroom during a therapeutic
m. The therapist should also be sensitive to the residents' feelings about incontinence and
the psychosocial consequences.

ons K/L. Oral/Nutritional Status and Oral/Dental Status

tion

many reasons for the decline of the ability to smell with age. For every 22 years we are
lose about half of our sensitivity to scents (Amoore, 1971). In addition, damage to the
al nerve, trauma, tumors, or infections near the olfactory nerve bulb can interfere with
to smell (Maloney, 1987). Those clients with a history of smoking have an increased
oss.

ntions Using Smell

an increase alertness in clients, the sense of smell can be useful to therapists. Histori-
ency personnel have used smelling salts to awaken a person who has lost conscious-
is a neurological basis for using olfactory stimulation (Ayres, 1978). Stimulation of
system leads to a connection in the midbrain called the reticular activating system.
eads to an arousal and central nervous system activation.
hat this type of stimulation can elicit strong emotions and memories in clients
; Farber, 1978). It is important to plan this intervention carefully, observe reactions,
o modify the activity accordingly.
mended that the odors used be related to the activity you have planned. Simply
veral vials of scents is not an appropriate therapeutic use of olfactory stimulation.
e, Mr. B. and Mrs. L. were usually inactive in cooking group until the very end of
en everyone sampled the food. It was difficult to get either resident to help in the
se of the program. Mr. B. was drowsy and refused to assist in opening, washing,
redients. Mrs. L. seemed confused, and she hoarded objects and ingredients in her
rapist decided to try a new approach with these two clients. She brought Mr. B.
e program 5 minutes early. Before the cooking group began she used cinnamon,
lla as a stimulus. Mr. B. was reminded of making cookies during the holidays for
. L. talked about her famous apple muffins, and all the ingredients needed to
residents were alert and more willing to help in the meal preparation group. Mr.
e stirring jobs, and Mrs. L. enjoyed peeling fresh fruit.
asily incorporated into treatment programs are fresh flowers, evergreens, fresh
. Peeling an orange before a program about vacations is a simple and wonder-
dents to remember trips to Florida. Remember, to be effective, an odor must
vely by the resident (Farber, 1978). Precautions should be taken not to irritate
xtra care using scents with residents with breathing disorders. Contact medical

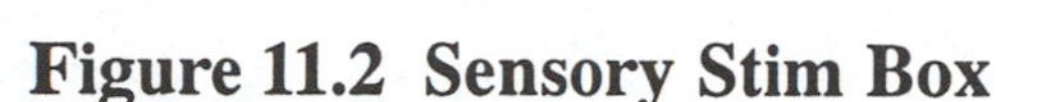

Figure 11.2 Sensory Stim Box

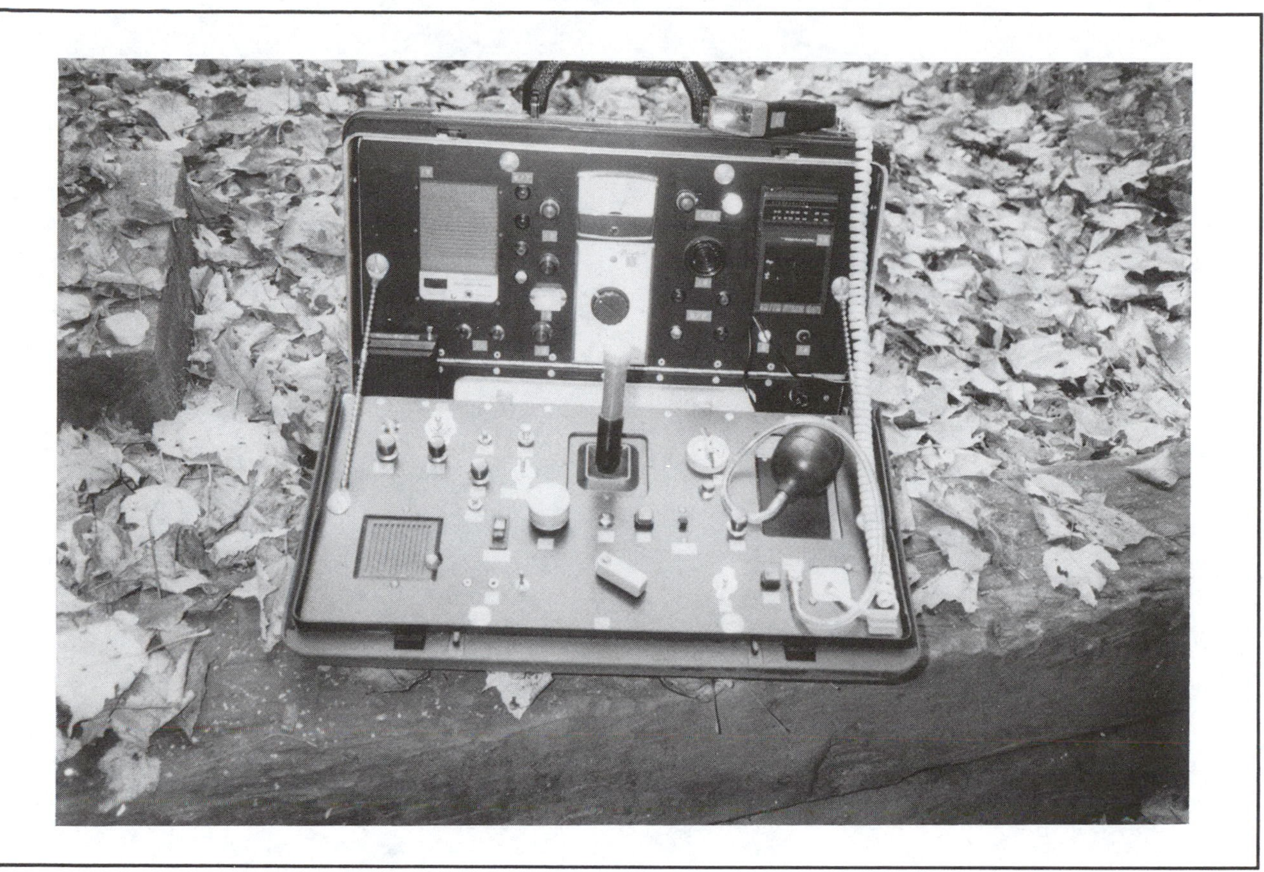

Chapter Twelve

The MDS and Continence, Oral/Nu
Status, Dental Status, and Skin Co

Section H. Continence

Incontinence is a major problem for nursing home residents and for th
estimated that over 50 percent of residents have incontinence episode
Dept. of Health and Human Services Clinical Guidelines: Urinary ir

There are many different types of incontinence. Urge incontiner
urine as soon as the need is felt. If a resident has urge incontinence
the bathroom quickly enough, need to urinate whenever she drinks
to the bathroom very often.

Stress incontinence causes the resident to leak urine when sne
The resident may have leakage occur when getting up from a cha
flow incontinence causes the resident to feel that the bladder is r
resident with this type of incontinence may go to the bathroom
for a long time, but doesn't urinate.

SECTION H. CONTINENCE IN LAST 14 DAYS			
1.	CONTINENCE SELF-CONTROL CATEGORIES *(Code for resident's PERFORMANCE OVER ALL S* 0. *CONTINENT*—Complete control *(includes use of indv or ostomy device that does not leak urine or stool)* 1. *USUALLY CONTINENT*—BLADDER, incontinent epis less; BOWEL, less than weekly 2. *OCCASIONALLY INCONTINENT*—BLADDER, 2 or m not daily; BOWEL, once a week 3. *FREQUENTLY INCONTINENT*—BLADDER, tended but some control present (e.g., on day shift); BOV 4. *INCONTINENT*—Had inadequate control. BLADDE BOWEL, all (or almost all) of the time		
a.	BOWEL CONTI-NENCE	Control of bowel movement, with ap continence programs, if employed	
b.	BLADDER CONTI-NENCE	Control of urinary bladder function (if d cient to soak through underpants), wit or continence programs, if employed	
2.	BOWEL ELIMIN-ATION PATTERN	Bowel elimination pattern regular—at least one movement every three days	a.
		Constipation 17*	b.
3.	APPLIANCES AND PROGRAMS	Any scheduled toileting plan	a.
		Bladder retraining program	b.
		External (condom) catheter 6	c.
		Indwelling catheter 6	d.
		Intermittent catheter 6	e.
4.	CHANGE IN URINARY CONTI-NENCE	Resident's urinary contin status of 90 days ago (c if less than 90 days) 0. No change 1.	

Reprinted with permission of Brig
Iowa 50306 • (800) 247-2343

that r
reside
progra
realize

Secti

Olfac

There ar
alive we
first crani
our ability
olfactory

Interve

Because it
cally, emerg
ness. There
the olfactory
This system
Be aware
(Moore, 1976
and be ready
It is recom
bringing out se
For examp
the program w
preparation pha
or chopping ing
pockets. The th
and Mrs. L. to th
nutmeg, and van
his children. Mrs
make them. Both
B. took over all th
Other stimuli
fruits or vegetable
ful way to help res
be perceived positi
the mucosa. Take

personnel if irregularities in breathing occur during your program. Artificial odors are generally not as effective as natural ones and sometimes have irritating ingredients.

Gustatory

Throughout life taste receptor cells wear out and are replaced. In older adults, the replacement rate slows down resulting in a weaker sense of taste (Maloney, 1987). The sweet taste receptors are the last ones to be affected in this process (Colavita, 1978). Thus, many older persons prefer sweet foods. This decrease in taste also explains why many older adults have poor appetites, and inadequate nutrition.

Interventions

The recreation therapist can be of great assistance at mealtime and with general nutrition. The therapist can discuss tastes and textures of foods while reminiscing with residents. The activities staff is often involved in outings that involve meals, or parties at which refreshments are served. In these settings it is important to compensate for decreased ability to perceive tastes.

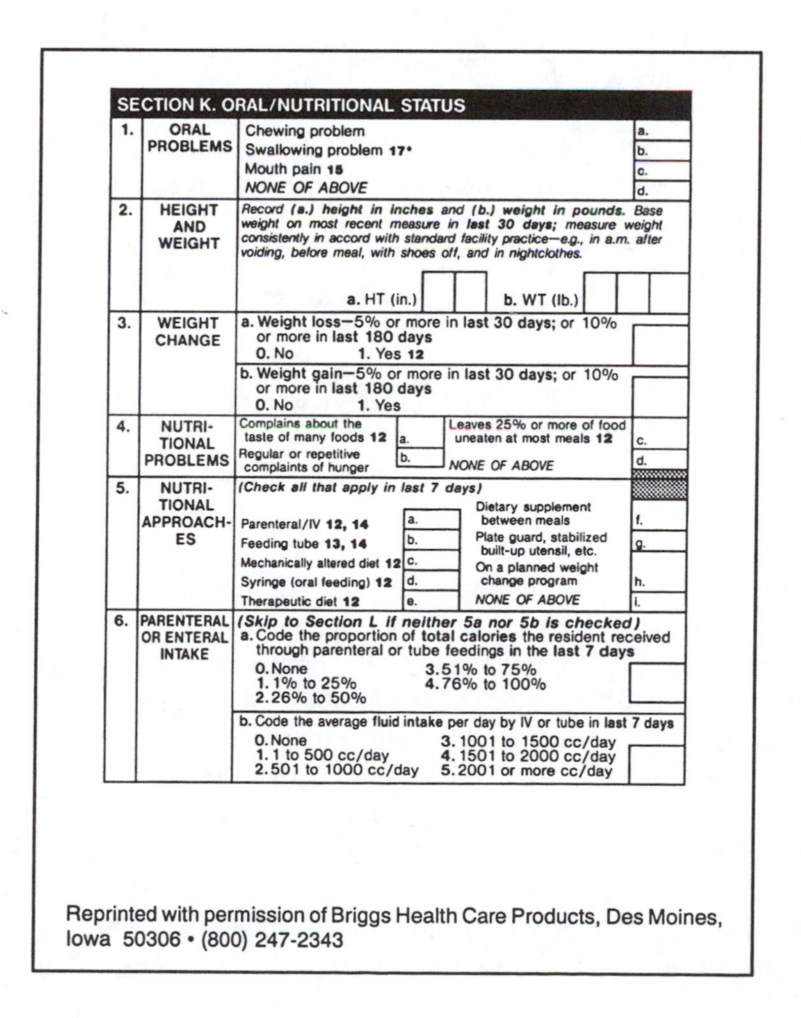

SECTION K. ORAL/NUTRITIONAL STATUS		
1.	ORAL PROBLEMS	Chewing problem a. Swallowing problem **17*** b. Mouth pain **15** c. *NONE OF ABOVE* d.
2.	HEIGHT AND WEIGHT	*Record (a.) height in inches and (b.) weight in pounds. Base weight on most recent measure in last 30 days; measure weight consistently in accord with standard facility practice—e.g., in a.m. after voiding, before meal, with shoes off, and in nightclothes.* a. HT (in.) b. WT (lb.)
3.	WEIGHT CHANGE	a. Weight loss—5% or more in last 30 days; or 10% or more in last 180 days 0. No 1. Yes **12** b. Weight gain—5% or more in last 30 days; or 10% or more in last 180 days 0. No 1. Yes
4.	NUTRITIONAL PROBLEMS	Complains about the taste of many foods **12** a. Regular or repetitive complaints of hunger b. Leaves 25% or more of food uneaten at most meals **12** c. *NONE OF ABOVE* d.
5.	NUTRITIONAL APPROACHES	*(Check all that apply in last 7 days)* Parenteral/IV **12, 14** a. Feeding tube **13, 14** b. Mechanically altered diet **12** c. Syringe (oral feeding) **12** d. Therapeutic diet **12** e. Dietary supplement between meals f. Plate guard, stabilized built-up utensil, etc. g. On a planned weight change program h. *NONE OF ABOVE* i.
6.	PARENTERAL OR ENTERAL INTAKE	*(Skip to Section L if neither 5a nor 5b is checked)* a. Code the proportion of total calories the resident received through parenteral or tube feedings in the last 7 days 0. None 1. 1% to 25% 2. 26% to 50% 3. 51% to 75% 4. 76% to 100% b. Code the average fluid intake per day by IV or tube in last 7 days 0. None 1. 1 to 500 cc/day 2. 501 to 1000 cc/day 3. 1001 to 1500 cc/day 4. 1501 to 2000 cc/day 5. 2001 or more cc/day

Reprinted with permission of Briggs Health Care Products, Des Moines, Iowa 50306 • (800) 247-2343

One idea is to use condiments to add extra flavor. Many facilities provide flavor enhancing spices on each dining room table. Watch out for the resident who adds 10 packets of sugar to her coffee or the entire contents of the salt shaker to her soup. There are serious health implications that may follow.

It is a good idea to provide finger foods at parties and special events. Many residents go without because they cannot maneuver a plate of cake and ice cream with a cup of tea. It is not dignified for the resident to be spoon fed in this setting, so why not serve foods that can be managed independently. Some suggestions include: ice cream cones or ice cream on a stick, a small cup cake or muffin, crackers and cheese, Jello jigglers, veggie sticks with dip, popcorn or pretzels, and cut up pieces of fresh fruit. Serve one thing at a time, and provide drinks to follow each serving of food.

Therapists must be vigilant concerning oral/dental status during programming involving food. Be sure residents are wearing their dentures before transporting them to programs. If a resident complains of any mouth discomfort notify nursing or medical staff immediately.

SECTION L. ORAL/DENTAL STATUS			
1.	ORAL STATUS AND DISEASE PREVEN-TION	Debris (soft, easily movable substances) present in mouth prior to going to bed at night **15**	a.
		Has dentures or removable bridge	b.
		Some/all natural teeth lost—does not have or does not use dentures (or partial plates) **15**	c.
		Broken, loose, or carious teeth **15**	d.
		Inflamed gums (gingiva); swollen or bleeding gums; oral abscesses; ulcers or rashes **15**	e.
		Daily cleaning of teeth/dentures or daily mouth care—by resident or staff Not ✓ - **15**	f.
		NONE OF ABOVE	g.

Reprinted with permission of Briggs Health Care Products, Des Moines, Iowa 50306 • (800) 247-2343

Section M. Skin

Touch/Proprioception

Touch and proprioception are important senses to utilize during therapeutic activities. Proprioception is the awareness of one's movements and position in space. For example, proprioception gives a resident a sense that she is bending or straightening a joint during an exercise group.

It is believed that a decreased elasticity of the skin leads to fewer touch receptor cells in older adults. It appears, however, that in many older adults that tactile perception remains relatively intact. That makes the sense of touch and the awareness of how the body is moving very important. This sense aids the older adult in self-care, even if he or she can not see things as well. Unimpaired tactile sense can also enable the older adult to continue former interests or take up new leisure skills.

When using touch as a technique, always alert the resident in another way first. Ask permission, use body language, eye contact, or demonstration before touching a resident. Ethnic customs and individual preferences must be considered. Although some residents crave touch, others may not be receptive to it.

Touch can be used in different ways. For example, light touch is often used at the beginning of a program to alert or stimulate the resident. Pressure touch is calming or reassuring. It is often used during the later stages of integrative group therapy or during closure of a session.

Touching objects or materials can be satisfying, especially for residents with dementia. A recommended approach is to use opposite materials. Some examples include: a dry wash cloth and a warm wet wash cloth, a sandpaper block and a smooth wood block, a piece of burlap and a piece of velvet. Sand, leather, kitchen utensils, heavy socks, large sea shells, and feathers are other objects to include in a touch kit.

It appears from the literature that movement and active tasks can lead to successful programs for older adults. A maximum use of proprioception and touch can be found in these programs. The recreation therapist or activities director in a long-term care facility must be aware of all these changes, and plan care and programs to match these aspects of each individual's life.

SECTION M. SKIN CONDITION

1.	**ULCERS** (Due to any cause)	*(Record the number of ulcers at each ulcer stage—regardless of cause. If none present at a stage, record "0" (zero). Code all that apply during* **last 7 days.** *Code 9 = 9 or more.) [Requires full body exam.]*	Number at Stage
		a. Stage 1. A persistent area of skin redness (without a break in the skin) that does not disappear when pressure is relieved.	
		b. Stage 2. A partial thickness loss of skin layers that presents clinically as an abrasion, blister, or shallow crater.	
		c. Stage 3. A full thickness of skin is lost, exposing the subcutaneous tissues—presents as a deep crater with or without undermining adjacent tissue.	
		d. Stage 4. A full thickness of skin and subcutaneous tissue is lost, exposing muscle or bone.	
2.	**TYPE OF ULCER**	*(For each type of ulcer, code for the* **highest stage in the last 7 days** *using scale in item M1—i.e., 0=none; stages 1, 2, 3, 4)*	
		a. Pressure ulcer—any lesion caused by pressure resulting in damage of underlying tissue 1 - **16**; 2, 3, or 4 - **12, 16**	
		b. Stasis ulcer—open lesion caused by poor circulation in the lower extremities	
3.	**HISTORY OF RESOLVED ULCERS**	Resident had an ulcer that was resolved or cured in **LAST 90 DAYS** 0. No 1. Yes **16**	
4.	**OTHER SKIN PROBLEMS OR LESIONS PRESENT**	*(Check all that apply during last 7 days)*	
		Abrasions, bruises	a.
		Burns (second or third degree)	b.
		Open lesions other than ulcers, rashes, cuts (e.g., cancer lesions)	c.
		Rashes—e.g., intertrigo, eczema, drug rash, heat rash, herpes zoster	d.
		Skin desensitized to pain or pressure **16**	e.
		Skin tears or cuts (other than surgery)	f.
		Surgical wounds	g.
		NONE OF ABOVE	h.
5.	**SKIN TREATMENTS**	*(Check all that apply during last 7 days)*	
		Pressure relieving device(s) for chair	a.
		Pressure relieving device(s) for bed	b.
		Turning/repositioning program	c.
		Nutrition or hydration intervention to manage skin problems	d.
		Ulcer care	e.
		Surgical wound care	f.
		Application of dressings (with or without topical medications) other than to feet	g.
		Application of ointments/medications (other than to feet)	h.
		Other preventative or protective skin care (other than to feet)	i.
		NONE OF ABOVE	j.
6.	**FOOT PROBLEMS AND CARE**	*(Check all that apply during last 7 days)*	
		Resident has one or more foot problems—e.g., corns, calluses, bunions, hammer toes, overlapping toes, pain, structural problems	a.
		Infection of the foot—e.g., cellulitis, purulent drainage	b.
		Open lesions on the foot	c.
		Nails/calluses trimmed during **last 90 days**	d.
		Received preventative or protective foot care (e.g., used special shoes, inserts, pads, toe separators)	e.
		Application of dressings (with or without topical medications)	f.
		NONE OF ABOVE	g.

Reprinted with permission of Briggs Health Care Products, Des Moines, Iowa 50306 • (800) 247-2343

Chapter Thirteen
Group Work

Bowlby (1992) defines a group as people "coming together with others with similar interests, needs, and capabilities" (p. 97). Program planning for a group requires a therapist to examine the special considerations of the group, format structure, and the leadership style necessary for success (Farrell & Lundegren, 1991). This chapter examines some of the facilitation techniques and group programs with proven efficacy in the nursing home setting.

Sensory Stimulation

Sensoristasis is the level of sensory information necessary for alertness and normal brain functioning. If there is too little, too much, or if the information is too complex, behavior becomes disorganized. Sensory stimulation is a program to help residents to maintain sensoristasis.

Sensory stimulation is often provided to residents who are bed patients and do not have the opportunity to seek out stimulation in the environment. The therapist usually provides a program of stimulation directed at all five senses in a one-to-one or small group setting. The actual activities range from kinesthetic awareness exercises to tasting and smelling activities. Visual stimulation often entails the use of brightly colored objects and mirrors. The goal of this therapy is to improve the resident's perception and alertness in response to the environment.

Care must be taken so that this does not become a program of sensory bombardment. Encouraging the resident to provide her own stimulation can help. She will generally select the sensory objects that are meaningful and pleasant. She will know when she has had enough.

A meaningful way to provide sensory stimulation is to help residents "get ready" for mealtime. A container of warm water, some scented soap, and a wet washcloth provide pleasant stimulation, and the resident should be encouraged to wash her own hands and face.

Room-based sensory stimulation programs can result in isolation for the resident. A therapist may visit for 15 minutes three times a week, but the resident is still alone for many hours of the day. Integrative group therapy may be more appropriate for some to prevent social isolation.

Sensory Stimulation Through Integrative Group Therapy

Instead of providing individual sensory stimulation in a resident's room, the therapeutic approach developed by Ross (1981, 1991) is an alternative technique. Ross's (1991) approach is based on neurophysiological principles and is provided in small groups. The integrative group process allows for socialization not just sensory stimulation. The stimulation is interesting and meaningful and is presented in a specific sequence.

Integrative group therapy has five stages. All five of the stages should be presented in each session to achieve the full benefit for each resident. In Stage 1 the therapist uses as many senses as possible to welcome and arouse the participants. In Stage 2 the resident is encouraged to move.

Stage 3 uses a variety of activities that offer an opportunity for modification. Through this modification the activities lead to meaningful adapted responses. Stage 4 activities help the resident produce organized thoughts and behaviors. Finally, in Stage 5, familiar activities culminate the session.

The therapist is constantly moving from resident to resident in this group therapy. She must make eye contact, use touch, and a calm voice with each resident. Residents are encouraged to provide their own stimulation and to interact with others in the group.

The criteria developed by Ross to evaluate the effectiveness of each treatment session includes the following:

1. Each group member will demonstrate acceptable behavior during each session.
2. Each participant will participate in at least one activity.
3. At the end of the session, the prevailing mood should be an alert calmness (Ross, 1991, p. 3).

Reminiscence

Examining one's past experiences is considered an essential human need (Butler, 1961). Some therapists believe that reminiscence is crucial to the emotional livelihood of older adults (Lieberman & Tobin, 1983). Careful planning should be done to assist residents to remember past experiences. Unresolved conflicts may come up, and the therapist can assist in successful reintegration. This process can help the older person add significance to her life and prepare for death. Memoirs, art, music, and objects from the past can be used to facilitate this process. The recreation therapist should be aware, however, that reminiscence can bring up painful experiences that may require the services of a mental health professional to assist the resident in the healing process.

Reality Orientation

Reality orientation is a specific set of techniques for assisting older adults with cognitive impairments to remain oriented and communicative. It was developed by James Folsom in 1958 and has been widely used in nursing homes. The program entails presenting residents who have severe impairments with simple, straight forward information on a regular basis by those who are caring for them. Residents with less severe impairments are provided with classes in which information is presented over and over. It may include information about the resident's name, current address, the date or season. Residents are encouraged to verbalize during the session.

Efficacy studies are inconclusive. The benefits of reality orientation programming seem to be small and of short duration (Reisberg, 1987). MacNeil and Teague (1987) have suggested that TR specialists should incorporate reality orientation techniques in their programs. This can be accomplished by briefly repeating who the therapist and resident are before starting the activity. Reviewing the program and the activities that have recently taken place, and highlighting daily programs to be held each morning in a one-to-one visit with confused residents are ways to incorporate reality orientation into a program.

Leisure Education

At a time of life when personal independence is important, many older adults in nursing homes feel alone and dependent on others. The use of wheelchairs, walkers, or gerichairs, coupled with incontinence and confusion, may isolate residents even more.

Family members and nurses aides often want to show they "care" and do more for the resident than is necessary. Family members may visit at a time when social/leisure skill sessions are taking place. Others might not want their family member to interact with peers who seem "worse off." The lack of nursing home staff to transport residents to and from programs is another problem that limits the resident.

The results of these experiences may reinforce dependency needs and diminish the residents' sense of control. When the resident learns that he or she is helpless in one situation, other behaviors may be negatively affected as well.

Many leisure researchers feel that helplessness occurs in people with disabilities because they do not have opportunities to demonstrate self-determined behaviors and personal control (Zoerink, 1988). Leisure education services, modified for older adults in long-term care settings, may help alleviate the effects of social isolation and learned helplessness (Iso-Ahola, MacNeil & Szymanski, 1980; Mundy & Odum, 1979).

The leisure education program should help residents: 1) identify recreation that is within his or her environment, 2) learn skills needed to find and use the recreational opportunities independently, 3) teach residents the options available on and off the residential unit, 4) discuss leisure patterns and priorities, 5) overcome barriers to participation in leisure time activities.

The recreation therapist needs to be creative in his or her leisure education approach, especially if residents have cognitive impairments. Integrating leisure skills into the daily routine is useful and often more meaningful. For example, the resident has verbalized an interest in photography but does not want to attend any classes. Just before a family visit is about to end or during a unit special event a camera and film can be made available. The therapist can show the resident how to load the camera and encourage her to shoot a few pictures of the situation.

Other simple ways to educate residents about leisure opportunities are to use small group projects. A crafts group can make and hang up large identifying signs for recreational sites. Residents in a cognitive therapy program might develop a choice board with colorful pictures and words describing recreational activities. During a joint program with the speech therapist the goal might be to improve the residents' ability to ask about locations or opportunities for recreation. By placing recreational materials all around the residential unit the therapist can increase leisure options. Signs with simple instructions placed over the activity at convenient locations where residents with dementia wander can allow for choice and experimentation.

Art as Group Therapy

Art is a form of behavior therapy. It can provide a useful way to fight disuse, decrease isolation, and facilitate communication. Art activities may enhance interactions between residents, residents and staff, and residents and families. Art can provide a balance between anxiety and boredom. It contributes to the growth of self and returns control to the individual. It can help an older individual find meaning in his or her existence (Sherritt & Pokorny, 1994).

An important concept to remember is that art activities should be used to facilitate meaningful leisure experiences. Emphasis should be on the process not the product. It should have nothing to do with the craft bazaar the facility puts on to raise money. This is therapy. The therapist's role is to facilitate involvement in an experience that is enjoyable and beneficial to the resident.

Animal Assisted Group Therapy

In animal assisted activities (AAA) a pet owner and his or her animal visit informally with hospital patients, nursing home residents, and people with disabilities. The animal assisted therapy (AAT) program has a more formal involvement with the treatment plan of the patient or resident.

There are training and registration programs for animal-people teams to complete health and temperament screening and training. This process assures that only well-trained therapists/volunteers and animals will be entering healthcare facilities. It is important to develop a policies and procedures document for the facilities' animal related programs.

There are many benefits of animal assisted therapy. Animals can help residents relax, concentrate, and focus on the moment. Research has shown there is a general increase in physical and emotional well-being in residents who bond with a pet. Many individuals also exhibit improved physical and cognitive functioning when involved with an animal.

Residents' responses that can be documented include:

1. Looks at pet,
2. Touches pet,
3. Speaks to pet,
4. Remembers pet's name,
5. Uses the pet's name,
6. Engages in activity with pet (e.g., walking, teaching tricks, combing or brushing),
7. Looks at therapist,
8. Speaks to therapist, and
9. Remembers therapist's name.

See Resources, page 141, for contact information on the Delta Society and the Pet Partners Program.

The Horticulture Group as Therapy

Keeping and caring for plants is a familiar pastime for many older people. It is rewarding to nurture and watch something grow. Working with plants is a lifetime skill that is often maintained, even in residents who have dementia.

Horticulture therapy can help bridge the gap between residents' protected environment and the "real" world. The needs of plants are similar to the needs of people. Without care and attention, both will fail to thrive. Individuals who are withdrawn can learn to relate to plants and then get involved more closely with other people doing the same thing. People love to talk about their gardens!

A horticulture program can be established for any resident who is interested. If a resident can get out-of-doors and work in a regular garden bed the program may simply involve making some short handled tools for people gardening from chairs. Eventually, raised beds can be built for those residents who cannot reach down to the ground. The greenhouses, tool sheds, and pathways all should be made accessible for wheelchairs.

Residents confined to beds can also garden. A recreation therapist can provide these residents with plastic sheets, a lapboard, and the plant materials. A mobile gardening cart stocked with planting materials can be used to increase interest levels of residents who do not want to go to the garden site.

Gardening in containers and window boxes provides an outlet for those who wish to garden indoors. If a facility does not have much space, bonsai gardening can be tried. The art of bonsai gardening can provide an interesting program in which miniature landscapes are created in shallow containers.

The gardening program can link individuals to other programs and people. For example, if residents grow vegetables, the harvest may yield a bounty for the cooking groups. The gardeners can harvest the crop of tomatoes, and the cooking group might make Gazpacho for everyone.

If herbs are grown, it is fun to dry some of the branches. The dried herbs can then be used to make tea to be bagged. Residents may then enjoy inviting family and friends to a tea social on a Sunday afternoon in the fall.

See Resources, page 141, for contact information on other horticulture/gardening ideas.

Section Four

Evaluation

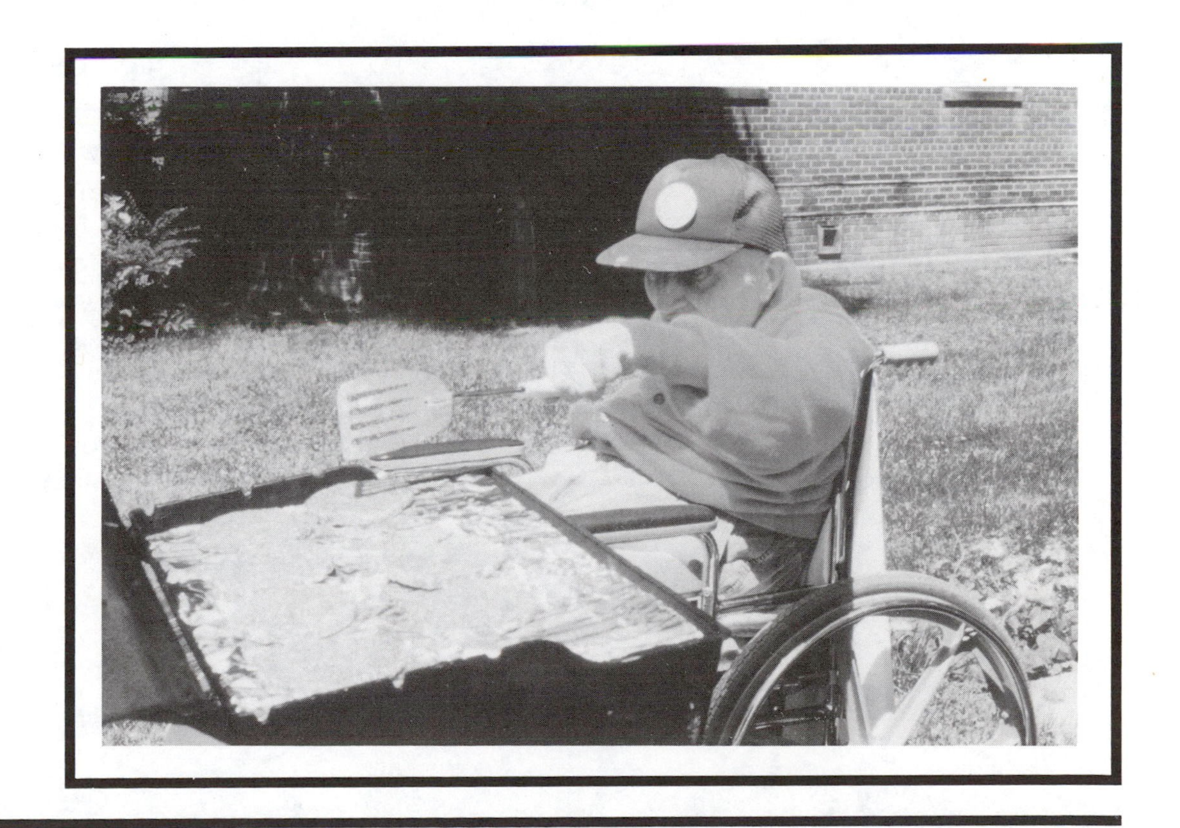

Chapter Fourteen
Documenting Progress

Documenting progress begins with assessment and continues on through treatment planning, treatment, and discharge. Good documentation tells other readers what the resident has done in recreation therapy, and how he or she did it:

1. Start with a thorough assessment of each resident. The MDS may not allow for enough information about the resident. Select other evaluation tools to use with the resident to make the outcome meaningful and measurable.
2. Develop a list of current skills and weakness areas. Note the resident's scores on evaluation instruments.
3. Prioritize the weakness areas. Take the most important area first and develop a goal which is attainable in the next few months.
4. Develop a plan of recreation therapy programs to attain the goal.
5. Develop a flow chart to document attendance in programs and the behaviors the resident exhibits in each session. See Appendix C for a sample.
6. Document the behaviors and progress toward the goal in the 90-day or 30-day note (new admission). Include the following in the note:

    - name the specific programs the resident attended;
    - the length of time in each program the resident was active;
    - what active things the resident did;
    - what activities the resident initiated;
    - what passive things the resident did;
    - was the resident alert or confused;
    - did the resident verbalize or make choices known;
    - did the resident interact socially with peers or staff;
    - level of socialization;
    - was the resident calm during and at the end of the program;
    - if not calm, what specific behaviors were seen and what triggered the behavior;
    - did the resident independently walk or wheel to and from the program—what distance was covered;
    - attainment or progress toward goals; and
    - future treatment recommendations.

See Figure 14.1, page 120, for a summary of general guidelines.

Example: A Case Study of Mrs. G.

Mrs. G. was admitted to the nursing home on 3/10/95 with a diagnosis of acute pulmonary edema and congestive heart failure. Her secondary diagnosis was multi-infarct dementia. She was depressed, and had stopped eating soon after her admission. She was described as "lethargic and

Figure 14.1. Summary of General Documentation Guidelines

1. All progress notes and care plans should be signed and dated by the TR staff who wrote the note.
2. Always write on the medical record in black ink unless another color code is specified for specific remarks.
3. Avoid generalizations or interpretations, like "confused" or "agitated." Instead, describe the actual behaviors that were observed.
4. Include rationale for your decisions and recommendations.
5. Include comments made by the resident and/or her family.
6. Never erase or use white-out if an error is made. Simply draw a line through the error and initial and date it.
7. If you are referring to material that appears elsewhere in the chart, refer to it by name, and tell where it is located.
8. Remember that one of the main purposes of documentation is to communicate with other healthcare professionals, so avoid using jargon or terms or abbreviations that others will not understand.
9. Be concise, but thorough, in the documentation. Remember that if it isn't written, it didn't happen. So, be sure to include all necessary information.

refusing to do anything" by her nurse. She was increasingly confused, awake all night, and sleeping late into the daytime hours. During the previous month Mrs. G. told several staff members that she was ready to die. She refused to leave her room and was spoon fed her meals at her bedside by nurses. She seemed increasingly weak and had been found on the floor near her bed on five occasions during the past month. Mrs. G. did not attend any group programs, but was visited every other day by activities staff for sensory stimulation.

Beyond the MDS Mrs. G. was assessed for strength using a bulb-type hand dynamometer, functioning using the M.O.S.E.S., and the Mini Mental State for cognitive functioning.

Scores documented:

Two lbs. bilaterally on the hand dynamometer (poor overall strength)

M.O.S.E.S.—Physical mobility problems
- Cognitive loss
- Sadness and depression
- Failure to respond to social contacts

Mini Mental State—score of 9 (serious cognitive impairment)

Strengths to work with: can make choices and is verbal, can follow simple directions, limited strength, seems to want to get out of bed at times.

Problem areas: depressed, isolated—no friends in the nursing home, poor strength and mobility, dependent on others for all personal care, no interests or desire to attend programs, at very high risk for falls.

Program direction: one-to-one sensory air flow mat therapy for strength, independence, and to develop a therapeutic relationship.

Leisure Education: to increase opportunities for friendships to develop and for independence in leisure.

Long-Range Goals:
- Mrs. G. will improve her strength.
- Mrs. G. will independently leave her room and use the leisure lounge activities daily.
- Mrs. G. will interact socially with staff and peers in the nursing home.

Short-Term Objectives:
- Mrs. G. will show trust in the recreation therapist as evidenced by going to the air mat therapy program when asked two times per week.
- Mrs. G. will transfer with assistance of her therapist onto the air mat using a safe one-person transfer.
- Mrs. G. will sit next to her therapist on the air mat with her feet on the floor for two to three minutes before being assisted further onto the mat.
- Mrs. G. will allow her therapist to assist her in an active assistive exercise routine for 10 minutes while on the air mat.
- Mrs. G. will relax for 5 minutes on the air mat and talk to her therapist.
- Mrs. G. will become aware of the location of the leisure lounge as she returns to her room (two doors down from her room).

Progress Note: Mrs. G. was assessed on 3/12/95 for strength, overall functioning, and mental status. The following problem areas were identified: poor strength and mobility, no interest or desire to attend programs or socialize, sad and depressed mood, at high risk for falls, and dependent on others.

Mrs. G. was scheduled for sensory air mat therapy two times a week for 30 minutes a session. She was sleeping in her gerichair when this therapist attempted to pick her up for the first session. When aroused and asked to attend she mumbled "I don't care." She was wheeled to the program area about 75 feet down the hallway. Mrs. G. was provided with sensory alertness stimulation in the form of massage to her hands and feet to gain her attention, and then assisted to transfer to the air mat by two staff members. She was confused at first, but was reminded that she was there for her therapy program. Mrs. G. was able to sit next to her therapist for 30 seconds at the edge of the air mat. She was passively assisted to a supported supine position on the mat, and provided with 5 minutes of upper extremity exercise with the therapy dowel. At the end of the 5 minutes Mrs. G. actively struck the therapy balloon 10 times back and forth with this therapist. She was encouraged to relax to finish the session. Mrs. G. said "I wish I had a bed like this in my room." She said her bed was uncomfortable, and she always woke up. She also talked briefly about her husband who had died, and what a good cook he was. Mrs. G. was calm and alert at the end of the first session. She interacted with this therapist appropriately. She was encouraged to note where the lounge was located as we returned to her room at the end of the session. She will continue to work on the objectives listed above for the next 30 days. Recommendations: increase sitting time on the edge of the air mat to 60 seconds in the next session; go into the leisure lounge to look around on return from the next program; gradually increase exercise time as tolerated over the next several sessions.

Methods for Monitoring Progress Toward Goals and Objectives

Different states and nursing homes within states vary in their method of record keeping. There are two main methods used for charting and documentation: source-oriented record keeping and problem-oriented record keeping. Whichever method is used, the therapeutic recreation department must be concerned with accurate and thorough documentation within that system.

In source-oriented record keeping each professional group documents separately from the other groups. Each group has its own section of the chart. It does not isolate and single out one client problem on which treatment is focused. Unfortunately, this method can result in overlapping, contradictory, or incomplete information about a resident. It does not promote interdisciplinary care and treatment of residents.

In problem-oriented record keeping, documentation and treatment is more coordinated. The chart is organized according to client problem areas rather than by discipline. The chart begins with a data base or initial assessments for the resident. A problem list is developed by one or more members of the treatment team. A care or treatment plan is designed based on the problems.

Chapter Fifteen
Quality Assurance

Quality Assurance (QA): Responding to Accountability

All healthcare providers have been asked to demonstrate quality. Not only must they prove quality exists but also they must show that it is cost-effective. To begin the process, quality services for therapeutic recreation must be defined.

What Does Quality Look Like?

Therapeutic recreation professionals must prove that the services they provide are beneficial to both the residents of long-term care and to the industry. Efficacy research, better assessments, and quality assurance (QA) which includes peer review will help in making healthcare providers more accountable.

According to the American Nurses Association, the ultimate purpose of QA in healthcare is to make certain that an agreed upon level of excellence is achieved in the delivery of services to consumers. The Joint Commission defines QA as a process that enables the health professional to identify areas of improvement, detect potential problem areas, and design strategies for overcoming deficient areas in patient care.

Bob Riley (1987) defines QA as "a process that sets the standards for performance, provides information about the achievement of those standards, and monitors whether improvement has taken place and the standards are being met" (p. 12). In essence, QA can assure that standards of acceptable professional behavior are met in long-term care (Riley, 1987).

Therefore, the ultimate purpose of QA in healthcare is to make certain that an agreed upon level of excellence is achieved in the delivery of services to the consumers. Basically, QA programs should be set up to evaluate therapeutic recreation practice.

JCAHO notes that the purpose of a QA program is to provide both a comprehensive format that is designed to ensure optimal patient/resident care using available resources and a program that is consistent with the achievable goals for the facility.

Riley (1987) breaks QA into two distinct yet interlocking systems to address these purposes, programmatic QA and global QA. The programmatic system includes staff review, peer review, client satisfaction, and QA programs developed at the facility. More globally, QA includes professional standards, accreditation, professional certification, and professional ethics. Global QA is established by professional organizations. Programmatic QA is set-up at individual nursing homes and hospitals. Ideally there is a feedback loop between programmatic and global QA if the true purpose is being met.

Written Plan of Operation

Before a recreation therapist can set up a quality assurance plan, a written plan of operation for both the facility and each department should be in place. This written plan is more than just a policy and procedure manual. It must be more descriptive of the actual clinical functioning of each department. There are two major types of written plans that concern those in therapeutic recreation.

The agency or facility plan of operation is prepared by the administrator with input from the department heads. Accreditation surveyors review these thoroughly. If therapeutic recreation is not included, surveyors won't look to therapeutic recreation as a major service of the nursing home. The agency or facility plan should include the following sections:

A. Patient management functions which include facility-wide procedures for intake, assessment, treatment plans, progress notes, and discharge summaries.
B. Program management which includes QA activities, patient care monitoring, staff growth and development, research activities, and patient rights.

The second type of plan is more unique to the specific departments of the nursing home. Therapeutic recreation is no exception.

The therapeutic recreation written plan of operation is prepared by the therapeutic recreation department. Any self-regulating professional therapeutic recreation department should have a comprehensive department-level written plan of operation. As accreditation standards become less prescriptive, each discipline needs to describe the profession's degree of accountability and contribution to quality of care.

According to Nancy Navar (1981) the following ideas must be addressed:

1. What is the philosophy of TR in the nursing home?
2. What are the overall goals of the nursing home's therapeutic recreation program?
3. What are the components of the comprehensive program? What programs fall into the treatment category—leisure education category, or recreation participation category?
4. How do clients become involved in each program component (e.g., referral, voluntary, or entrance criteria)?
5. What specific programs are provided?
6. How are specific programs evaluated? How often?
7. What are the types of client assessment used? When is it used? Who is qualified to perform assessments?
8. What policies, procedures, or forms are utilized by the therapeutic recreation department?
9. How does therapeutic recreation interact with other services at the nursing home? Interdisciplinary programs should be listed in this section of the written plan.
10. What is the role of therapeutic recreation in relation to patient management at the nursing home? Plan for intake, assessment, care plans, discharge and aftercare.
11. What is the role of therapeutic recreation in relation to program management functions—QA activities, staff development, research, resident rights?

These written plans are the building blocks of QA. They must be agency-specific and can be in loose-leaf notebooks or some other format that is easily amended.

Establishing QA Standards for Therapeutic Recreation

According to the JCAHO, there are four main steps to establishing quality assurance. First, the JCAHO expects that the staff who are planning the QA process are competent to do so. That means the individuals are professionally educated and have proper credentials in the field of therapeutic recreation.

Second, the professional staff should determine the most important aspects of resident care. Four to seven items are recommended. These often include assessment, involvement in treatment planning, accuracy in progress notes, and provision of a comprehensive program. For example, the program should include treatment, leisure education, and opportunities for independent recreation participation.

Third, the professional staff must determine objective criteria that will represent each of the important aspects of resident care. For example, progress notes should be timely and accurate.

Last, the professional staff or department head will determine how each item will be monitored. For example, bimonthly chart review by the department head will be used to determine if progress notes were timely and accurate.

Assessing Quality

Quality assessment is the process of collecting targeted data, and doing something with it. What can a therapeutic recreation specialist do with it? There are three basic actions needed:

1. Analyze and compare it against predetermined standards.
2. Take appropriate action to correct a problem.
3. Manage the entire review operation.

How can the therapist or department head gather and organize data?

1. Resident charts have been traditionally the richest source of information.
2. Recreation management systems which include numbers and types of services and programs conducted, attendance records, progress notes.
3. Institutional data systems such as results of agency-wide utilization reviews, readmission data, or incident reports.
4. Events, both positive and negative, can be a rich and valuable source of data for the therapist. Examples include incident reports of falls or missing documentation.
5. Staff meetings often reveal issues and concerns raised by staff. Staff can be an extremely important source of data.
6. Direct observation of programs provides clear evidence of quality or sometimes problems. Peer review and day-to-day observation by a supervisor can be very helpful.
7. Client surveys and interviews help the recreation therapy department get the consumer's perspective on services.
8. Research can produce valuable insights for the recreation therapy department. In-house research projects can lead to establishing many valid QA standards and sources of data.

For example, measuring residents' strength, flexibility, or ability to ambulate or wheel independently to programs every three months may indicate that more residents need a therapeutic exercise program. Measuring behaviors during programs and during non-program time may show that fewer behavior problems occur when residents are active and involved. These data may help justify hiring a another staff member to provide leisure education.

Analyzing the Information

After all data have been gathered, the recreation therapist must do something with it. The therapist should look at differences between his or her actual practices and preestablished norms. Then case-by-case he or she should make recommendations for improvements.

For example, a therapist knows there should be programming in the treatment, leisure education, and recreation participation areas. It is discovered that few residents are actually receiving any leisure education. Red flags should go up! There is a gap in services. It is recommended to the staff that each therapist revise their programming. Each staff member should establish one evening or weekend leisure education program with the goal of the residents' gradually assuming responsibility.

Information Use

Once a problem is identified through the analysis, timely and appropriate action must be taken to correct the "red flagged" situations. Some of the other strategies that might be used are: workshops or education in weak areas, staff changes, temporary additional help either paid or through volunteers, interdisciplinary programming.

In conclusion, even the best QA systems in therapeutic recreation have problems. The therapists with the highest percentages on QA measures at a long-term care facility might be most interested in just that—high percentages on paperwork. It is vital to remember that quality assurance is about the residents.

Chapter Sixteen
Certification

Certification is a type of credentialing. It is usually voluntary and does not prevent others from practicing in the profession. Certification does, however, prevent uncertified individuals from using the title. In the certification process a private agency attests to the competence of an individual and grants that individual the right to use the credential.

The National Certification Council for Activity Professionals (NCCAP) offers three levels of certification and either two or three tracks to become certified at each level. The academic track is one in which formal education beyond high school is the basis for certification. The equivalency track is an alternate route, combining academics and work experience. There is no requirement for an internship under a certified professional and no certification exam. Many different academic backgrounds are acceptable for this certification. There is no time limit on how long ago the academic work may have taken place. If one has NCCAP certification it does *not* mean that that person is a Certified Therapeutic Recreation Specialist (C.T.R.S.).

The National Council for Therapeutic Recreation Certification (NCTRC) certifies recreation therapists through a national certification examination. To be qualified to sit for the national certification exam the therapist must have at least a bachelors degree in recreation/leisure services and must have met specific coursework requirements in recreation therapy. In addition, a 400-hour internship under a C.T.R.S. is required. Candidates are then allowed to sit for the national certification exam. If a therapist passes the exam he or she is certified for a period of five years, and awarded the right to use the letters C.T.R.S. after his or her name. Recertification is required every five years. Recertification has three major components: professional experience, continuing education, and reexamination.

Activity Director Certified

The Activity Director Certified (ADC) is one who meets NCCAP standards to direct/coordinate/supervise an activity program, staff and department primarily in a geriatric setting.

Track 1	Track 2	Track 3
(A) Bachelors Degree (must include eight required coursework areas).	(A) 60 College semester units (2 years) including required coursework.	(A) 30 College semester units (1 year)
and	and	and
(B) 2,000 hours within past five years.	(B) 6,000 hours (3 years) experience	(B) 10,000 hours (five years experience)
and	and	and
(C) 30 Continuing Education clock hours	(C) 30 Continuing Education clock hours	(C) 30 Continuing Education clock hours

Reprint permission granted by Marilyn Jaeger, NCCAP administrator, 5/30/95

Activity Assistant Certified

The Activity Assistant Certified (AAC) is one who meets NCCAP standards to assist in carrying out, with supervision, an activity program.

Track 1

(A) 30 College semester credits (1 year) including required coursework

and

(B) 2,000 hours within past five years.

and

(C) 20 Continuing Education clock hours

Track 2

(A) High School Diploma or Equivalent

and

(B) Basic Activity Course or three College semester units

and

(C) 4,000 hours (2 years) experience

and

(D) 20 Continuing Education clock hours

Reprint permission granted by Marilyn Jaeger, NCCAP administrator, 5/30/95

NCTRC or C.T.R.S. Requirements

Track 1—Academic Path

Baccalaureate degree or higher from an accredited college/university including:

(A) 18 semester units of therapeutic recreation and general recreation coursework;

(B) 18 semester units from three of the following six areas: adaptive physical education, related biological/physical sciences, human services, psychology, sociology, or special education; and,

(C) 360 hours of supervised field placement experience.

Track 2—Equivalency Path

Baccalaureate degree or higher from an accredited college/university including:

(A) 18 semester units of therapeutic recreation and general recreation coursework at the upper division or graduate level;

(B) 24 semester units from three of the following six areas: adaptive physical education, related biological/physical sciences, human services, psychology, sociology, or special education; and,

(C) Five years of full-time, paid experience.

Reprint permission granted by Marilyn Jaeger, NCCAP administrator, 5/30/95

Chapter Seventeen
The Therapeutic Recreation Consultant

The most common function of a TR consultant in the nursing home is that of an outsider to help solve problems through a new perspective. This consultant can ask pertinent questions, may write reports with suggested answers, and can serve as a catalyst for change or as a role model for staff. The consultant, however, may be seen as a threat to insecure staff.

Using consultants as facilitators rather than experts can enable the nursing home to become its own investigator and the problem solver. This role may be less threatening because it allows the organization to be in charge of the planning process. The facilitator engages the staff closest to the problem in the opportunity to solve the problem. This method of consulting aims to combine the nursing home's assets with an external resource.

Why Hire a Consultant?

Survey teams are beginning to enforce the OBRA '87 regulation in regard to providing therapeutic recreation. Few nursing homes have a certified therapeutic recreation specialist on staff. The nursing home administrator may choose to contract with a C.T.R.S. consultant as the result of a poor survey. Some of the services the therapeutic recreation consultant can assist with include:

- Clinical interventions for difficult-to-program residents,
- Staff training,
- Establishing clinical protocols,
- Documentation efforts such as goal writing, charting, and the assessment process,
- Setting up quality assurance programs,
- Trouble shooting on specialized care units,
- Research projects,
- Providing contractual programs like Leisure Education, and
- Transition from an Activities Department to a Recreation Therapy Department.

What Should You Look for in a Consultant?

- At least a master's degree prepared therapist
- Extensive experience in gerontological settings
- C.T.R.S.

What Will It Cost?

Be prepared to pay a consultant $25 to $75 per hour. Some of the clinical services may be reimbursable.

Where Can You Find a Consultant if You Need One?

A local college or university that has a graduate program in Recreation Therapy may be able to recommend a consultant, or the survey team may be able to recommend a consultant. The ATRA (American Therapeutic Recreation Association) or NCTRC (National Council for Therapeutic Recreation Certification) may have listings for consultants in your area.

References

Aasen, N. (1987). Interventions to facilitate personal control. *Journal of Gerontological Nursing, 13*, 21-28.

American Psychiatric Association. (1980). *Diagnostic and statistical manual for mental disorders* (3rd ed.). Washington, DC.

Amoore, J. E. (1971). Olfactory genetics and anosmia. In L. M. Beidler (Ed.), *Handbook of sensory physiology*, IV, 1. New York, NY: Springer-Verlag New York, Inc.

Austin, D. R. (1991). *Therapeutic recreation: Process and techniques,* 2nd ed. Champaign, IL: Sagamore Publishing, Inc.

Avedon, E. M. (1974). *Therapeutic recreation service: An applied behavioral science approach.* Englewood Cliffs, NJ: Prentice-Hall.

Axline, V. M. (1969). *Play therapy* (rev. ed.). New York, NY: Ballentine Books.

Ayres, A. J. (1978). *Sensory integration and learning disorders*. Los Angeles, CA: Western Psychological Services.

Baack, S. A. (1985). Recreation program participation by older adults: Its relationship to perceived freedom in leisure and life satisfaction. *Dissertation Abstracts International, 47*, 158.

Baley, J. A. (1955). Recreation and the aging process. *Research Quarterly, 26*, 1-7.

Banzinger, G. and Roush, S. (1983). Nursing homes for the birds: A control-relevant intervention with bird feeders. *The Gerontologist, 23*(5), 527-531.

Bengtson, V. L. (1973). *The social psychology of aging*. Indianapolis, IN: Bobbs-Merril Company, Inc.

Birren, J., Sloane, R. B., and Cohen, G. (1992). *Handbook of Mental Health and Aging*. San Diego, CA: Academic Press, Inc.

Bjorksten, J. (1974). Cross-linkage and the aging process. In M. Rockstein (Ed.), *Theoretical aspects of aging* (p. 43). New York, NY: Academic Press.

Bosse, R. and Ekerdt, D. J. (1981). Change in self perception of leisure activities with retirement. *The Gerontologist, 21*, 650-654.

Bowker, L. H. (1982). *Humanizing institutions for the aged*. Lexington, MA: Lexington Books.

Bowlby, C. (1992). *Therapeutic activities with persons disabled by Alzheimer's disease and related disorders*. Gathersburg, MD: Aspen Publishers, Inc.

Buettner, L. (1988). Utilizing developmental theory and adapted equipment with regressed geriatric patients in therapeutic recreation. *Therapeutic Recreation Journal, 22*(3), 72-79.

Buettner, L. (1994). "Therapeutic recreation as an intervention for persons with dementia and agitation: An efficacy study." Unpublished Doctoral Thesis, University Park, PA: Pennsylvania State University.

Butler, R. N. (1961). Re-Awaking interest. *Nursing Homes, 10*, 8-19.

Butler, R. N. (1963). The lifereview: An interpretation of reminiscence in the aged. *Psychiatry, 26*, 65-76

Butler, R. and Lewis, N. (1982). *Aging and mental health: Positive psychosocial and biomedical approaches*. St. Louis, MO: The C. V. Mosby & Year Book Medical Publishers, Inc.

Carpenito, L. J. (1992). *Nursing diagnosis: Application to clinical practice,* 4th ed. Philadelphia, PA: J. B. Lippincott Company.

Cassell, E. J. (1974). Dying in a Technological Society. In P. Steinfels and R. M. Veatch (Eds.), *Death Inside Out: The Hastings Center Report* (pp. 43-48). New York, NY: Harper & Row, Publishers, Inc.

Cockerham, W. (1991). *This aging society*. Englewood Cliffs, NJ: Prentice-Hall, Inc.

Cohen-Mansfield, J. and Bellig, N. (1986). Agitated behaviors in the elderly. *Journal of American Geriatric Society, 34*, 711-721.

Colavita, F. B. (1978). *Sensory changes in the elderly*. Springfield, IL: Charles C. Thomas, Publisher.

Cormier, W. H. and Cormier, L. S. (1985). *Interviewing strategies for helpers*. Monterey, CA: Brooks/Cole Publishing Co.

Coulton, C. and Frost, A. K. (1982). Use of social and health services by the elderly. *Journal of Health and Human Development, 23*, 330-339.

Cowgill, D. O. and Baulch, N. (1962). The use of leisure time by older people. *The Gerontologist, 2*, 47-50.

Crawford, D. W. and Godbey, G. (1987). Reconceptualizing barriers to family leisure. *Leisure Sciences, 9,* 119-127.

Csikszentmihalyi, M. (1975). *Beyond boredom and anxiety*. San Francisco, CA: Jossey-Bass, Inc., Publishers.

Cumming, E. and Henry, W. (1961). *Growing old: The process of disengagement*. New York, NY: Basic Books, Inc.

Cunningham, D. A., Montoye, H. J., Metzer, H. L., and Keller, J. B. (1968). Active leisure time activities as related to age among mean in a total population. *Journal of Gerontology, 23*, 551-556.

Department of Health. (1989). Federal Register, *54*(21), 5316-5373.

Dattilo, J. and Smith, R. W. (1990). Communicating positive attitudes toward people with disabilities through sensitive terminology. *Therapeutic Recreation Journal, 24*, 8-17.

Doress, P. B. and Siegal, D. L. (1987). *Ourselves, growing older: Women aging with knowledge and power*. New York, NY: Simon & Schuster, Inc.

Eslinger, R. and Damasio, A. (1986). Perserved motor function in Alzheimer's disease: Implications for anatomy and behavior. *The Journal of Neuroscience, 6*(10), 3006-3009.

Farrell, P. and Lundegren, H. M. (1991). *The process of recreation programming theory and technique*, 3rd ed. State College, PA: Venture Publishing, Inc.

Ferrari, N. A. (1962). "Institutionalization and attitude change in an aged population: A field study and dissidence theory." Unpublished doctoral dissertation. Western Reserve University. Cited in S. E. Iso-Ahola, (1980), Perceived control and responsibility as mediators of the effects of therapeutic recreation on the institutionalized aged. *Therapeutic Recreation Journal, 1*, 36-43.

Focus on Geriatric Care and Rehabilitation, 1, Number 1, 1987.

Folstein, M. F., Folstein, S. E., and McHugh, P. R. (1975). Mini Mental State: A practical method for grading the cognitive state of patients for the clinician. *Journal of Psychiatry Research, 12*, 189-198.

Frye, V. and Peters, M. (1972). *Therapeutic recreation: Its theory, philosophy, and practice.* Harrisburg, PA: Stackpole Books.

Gazda, G. M., Asbury, F. S., Balzer, F. J., Childers, W. C. , and Walters, R. P. (1984). *Human relations development: A manual for educators*, (3rd ed.). Boston, MA: Allyn & Bacon, Inc.

German, P., Rovner, B., Burton, L., Brandt, L., and Clark, R. (1992). The role of mental morbidity in the nursing home experience. *The Gerontologist, 32*(2), 152-163.

Godbey, G., Patterson, A., and Szwak-Brown. (1982). Rethinking leisure services in an aging population. *Parks and Recreation, 17*, 46-48.

Goldstein, A. P. (1980). Relationship-enhancement methods. In F. H. Kanfer and A. P. Goldstein (Eds.), *Helping people change* (pp. 18-57). New York, NY: Pergamon Press, Inc.

Gordon, C., Gaitz, C. M., and Scott, J. (1976). *Leisure and lives: Personal expressivity across the lifespan. Handbook of aging and social sciences.* New York, NY: Van Nostrand Reinhold.

Gottesman, L. and Bourestom, N. (1974). Why nursing homes do what they do. *Gerontologist, 14*, 156-163.

Harmon, D. (1986). Free radical theory of aging. In J. E. Johnson, R. L. Walford, D. Harmon, and J. Miguel (Eds.), *Free radicals, aging, and degenerative diseases.* New York, NY: Alan R. Liss.

Havinghurst, R. (1963). Successful aging. In R. Williams, C. Tibbitts, and W. Donahue (Eds.), *Processes of aging.* New York, NY: Atherton.

Hayflick, L. (1966). Senescence and cultured cells. In N. Shock (Ed.), *Perspectives in experimental gerontology.* Springfield, IL: Charles C. Thomas Publisher.

Hayflick, L. (1983). Theories of aging. In R. Cape, R. Coe, and M. Rodstein (Eds.), *Fundamentals of geriatric medicine.* New York, NY: Raven Press.

Helmes, E., Csapo, K. G., and Short, J. A. (1987). Standardization and validation of the multidimensional observation scale for elderly subjects (MOSES). *Journal of Gerontology, 42*, 395-405.

Hoar, J. (1961). A study of free-time activities of 200 aged persons. *Sociology and Social Research, 45*, 157-163.

Hooker, K. and Ventis, D. (1984). Work Ethic, Daily Activites, and Retirement Satisfaction. *Journal of Gerontology, 39*, 478-484.

Howe-Murphy, R. and Charboneau, B. C. (1978). *Therapeutic recreation intervention: An ecological perspective.* Englewood Cliffs, NJ: Prentice-Hall, Inc.

Hulicka, I., Morganti, J., and Cataldo, J. (1975). Perceived latitude of choice of institutionalized and non-institutionalized elderly women. *Experimental Aging Research, 1*(1), 27-39.

International Review of Applied Psychology, 32(2), 153-181. (From Psyclit Database, 1988, Abstract No. 75-14496).

Iso-Ahola, S. E. (1980). Perceived control and responsibility as mediators of the effects of therapeutic recreation on the institutionalized aged. *Therapeutic Recreation Journal, 1*, 36-43.

Iso-Ahola, S. E., MacNeil, R. D., and Szymanski, O. J. (1980). Social psychological foundations of therapeutic recreation: An attributional analysis. In S. E. Iso-Ahola (Ed.), *Social psychological perspectives on leisure and recreation.* Springfield, IL: Charles C. Thomas, Publisher.

Jeffares, D. W. (1986). Freedom of choice and its relationship to happiness in a group of new residents in public housing for the elderly. *Dissertation Abstracts International, 47*, 2697.

Johnson, D. W. (1981). *Reaching out: Interpersonal effectiveness and self-actualization.* Englewood Cliffs, NJ: Prentice-Hall.

Joint Commission (JCAHO) (1994). *Standards and protocol for dementia special care units.* Oakbrook, IL: Joint Commission on Accreditation of Healthcare Organizations.

Kelly, J. R., Steinkamp, M. W., and Kelly, J. R. (1986). Later Life Leisure: How they play in Peoria. *The Gerontologist, 26*, 531-544.

Kemp, B. and Mitchell, J. (1992). Functional assessment in geriatric mental health. In J. Birren, R. B. Sloane, and G. Cohen, (1992), *Handbook of mental health and aging*, pp. 671-697. San Diego, CA: Academic Press.

Knudson, D. M. (1984). *Outdoor recreation*, 2nd ed. New York, NY: MacMillan Publishing Company.

Langer, E. J. and Rodin, J. (1976). The effects of choice and enhanced personal responsibility for the aged: A field experiment in an institutional setting. *Journal of Personality and Social Psychology, 34*, 191-198.

Lawton, M. P., Moss, M. and Fulcomer, M. (1986-87). Objective and subjective uses of time by older people. *International Journal of Aging and Human Development, 24*, 171-188.

Lefcourt, H. M. (1982). *Locus of control, current trends in theory and research,* 2nd ed. Hillsdale, NJ: Lawrence Erlbaum Associates, Inc.

Lieberman, M. and Tobin, S. (1983). *The experience of the old age: Stress, coping, and survival.* New York, NY: Basic Books, Inc.

Louis Harris and Associates (1975). In National Council on Aging: *The myth and reality of aging in America*. Washington, DC: National Council on Aging.

MacNeil, R. D. and Teague, M. (1987). *Aging and Leisure*: *Vitality in later life*. Englewood Cliffs, NJ: Prentice-Hall.

Maloney, C. (1987). Identifying and treating the client with sensory loss. Physical and Occupational Therapy in Geriatrics, 5(4), 31-46.

Mannell, R. C., Zuzanek, J., and Larson, R. (1988). Leisure states and 'flow' experiences: Testing perceived freedom and intrinsic motivation hypotheses. *Journal of Leisure Research*, *20*(4), 289-304.

Martin, S. and Smith, R. W. (1993). OBRA legislation and recreational activities: Enhancing personal control in nursing homes. *Activities, Adaptation & Aging*, *17*(3), 1-14.

Maslow, A. H. (1968). *Toward a psychology of being*, 2nd ed. New York, NY: Van Nostrand Reinhold.

McAvoy, L. H. (1977). Needs of the elderly: An overview of the research. *Parks and Recreation*, *12*, 31-55.

Miller, J. B. (1976). *Toward a new psychology of women,* 2nd ed. Boston, MA: Beacon Press.

Miller, W. R. and Rollnick, S. (1991). *Motivational interviewing*. New York, NY: The Guilford Press.

Mobily, K. (1982). Physical activity and aging. In M. L. Teague, R. D. MacNeil, and G. L. Hitzhusen (Eds.), *Perspectives on leisure and aging in a changing society* (p. 384-426). Columbia, MO: University of Missouri.

Moore, N. C. (1976). Is paranoid illness associated with sensory deficits in the elderly. *Journal of Psychosomatic and Research*, *25*, 69-74.

Morgan, A. and Godbey, G. (1978). The effect of entering an age-segregated environment upon the leisure activity patterns of older adults. *Journal of Leisure Research*, *10*, 177-190.

Moss, F. E. and Halamandaris, V. J. (1977). *Too old, too sick, too bad*: *Nursing homes in America*. Germantown, MD: Aspen Publishers, Inc.

Mundy, J. and Odum, L. (1979). *Leisure education*: *Theory and practice*. New York, NY: John Wiley & Sons, Inc.

Murphy, J. F. (1975). *Recreation and leisure services*. Dubuque, IA: William C. Brown Company, Publishers.

Myers, J. E. (1990). *Empowerment for later life*. Ann Arbor, MI: Eric Resources Information Center.

Nasar, J. L. and Farokhpay, M. (1985). Assessment of Activity Priorities and Design Preferences of Elderly Residents in Public Housing: A case study. *The Gerontologist*, *25*, 251-257.

National Outdoor Recreation Plans, In Knudson, (1984). *Outdoor recreation*, 2nd ed. New York, NY: MacMillan Publishing Company.

Navar, N. (1981). A study of professionalization of therapeutic recreation in the state of Michigan. *Therapeutic Recreation Journal, 15*(2), 50-56.

Neulinger, J. (1974). *The psychology of leisure,* 2nd ed. Springfield, IL: Charles C. Thomas, Publisher.

Neutgarten, B. L. (1975). *Middle age and aging*. Chicago, IL: University of Chicago Press.

Omnibus Reconciliation Act of 1987. Department of Health and Human Services: Health Care Financing Administration. (1989). Rules and Regulations. *Federal Register, 54*(21), 5316-5373.

Parsons, M. B., Reid, D. H., Reynolds, J., and Bumgarner, M. (1990). Effects of chosen versus assigned jobs on the work performance of persons with severe handicaps. *Journal of Applied Behavioral Analysis, 23*(2), 253-258.

Pennsylvania Department of Environmental Resources, (1991). *Recreation Participation Survey.* Pennsylvania State Data Center Institute of State and Regional Affairs, Penn State Harrisburg.

Peppers, L. G. (1976). Patterns of leisure and adjustment to retirement. *The Gerontologist, 16*, 441-446.

Peterson, C. A. and Gunn, S. L. (1984). *Therapeutic recreation program design: Principles and procedures*. Englewood Cliffs, NJ: Prentice-Hall, Inc.

Pfeiffer, E. and Davis, G. C. (1971). The use of leisure time in middle life. *The Gerontologist, 11*, 187-195.

Prochaska, J. O. and DiClemente, C. C. (1982). Transtheoretical therapy: Toward a more integrative model of change. Psychotherapy. *Theory Research, and Practice, 19*, 276-288.

Ragheb, M. G. and Griffith, C. A. (1982). The contribution of leisure participation and leisure satisfaction to life satisfaction of older persons. *Journal of Leisure Research, 14*, 295-306.

Realon, R. E., Favell, J. E., and Lowerre, A. (1990). The effects on making choices engagement levels with persons who are profoundly multiply handicapped. *Education and Training in Mental Retardation, 25*(3), 299-305.

Reisburg, B. (1987). Reality orientation. In G. Maddox (Ed.), *The encyclopedia of aging*, pp. 558-59. New York, NY: Springer Publishing Co.

Riley, B. (1987). *Evaluation of therapeutic recreation through quality assurance.* State College, PA: Venture Publishing, Inc.

Robertson, R. D. (1988). Recreation and the institutionalized elderly: Conceptualization of the free choice and intervention continuums. *Activities, Adaptation & Aging, 11*, 61-73. (From Psyclit Database, 1989, Abstract No. 76-20208).

Rodin, J. (1983). Behavioral medicine: Beneficial effects of self-control training in aging. *International Review of Applied Psychology, 32*(2), 153-181.

Rodin, J. and Langer, E. J. (1977). Long-term effects of a control-relevant intervention with the institutionalized aged. *Journal of Personality and Social Psychology, 35*, 897-902.

Rogers, C. R. (1957). The necessary and sufficient conditions of therapeutic personality change. *Journal of Consulting Psychology, 21*, 95-103.

Rogers, C. R. (1961). *On becoming a person: A therapist's view of psychotherapy*. Boston, MA: Houghton Mifflin Company.

Ross, M. (1991). *Integrative group therapy: The structured five-stage approach.* Thorofare, NJ: Slack Inc.

Ross, M., and Burdick, D. (1981). *Sensory integration: A training manual.* Thorofare, NJ: Slack Inc.

Russell, R. V. (1984). Correlates of life satisfaction in retirement. *Dissertation Abstracts International, 46*, 2808.

Schmitt, F. A., Logue, P. E., and Farber, J. F. (1988). Predicting intellectual functioning from mini-mental state examination. *Journal of the American Geriatric Society, 36*, 509-510.

Schulz, R. (1976). Effects of control and predictability on the physical and psychological well-being of the institutionalized aged. *Journal of Personality and Social Psychology, 33*, 563-573.

Schulz, R. and Hanusa, B. H. (1978). Long-term effects of control and predictability-enhancing interventions: Findings and ethical issues. *Journal of Personality and Social Psychology, 36*, 1194-1201.

Seligman, M. P. (1975). *Helplessness: On depression, development and death.* San Francisco, CA: W. H. Freeman & Co.

Shary, J. M. and Iso-Ahola, S. E. (1989). Effects of a control-relavant intervention on a nursing home residents' perceived competence and self-esteem. *Therapeutic Recreation Journal, 23*, 7-16.

Sherritt, P. and Pokorny, M. (1994). Art Activities for Patients with Alzheimer's and Related Disorders. *Geriatric Nursing, 15*(3), 155-159.

Sommer, R. and Osmond, H. (1960-61). Symptons of institutional care. *Social Problems, 8*(3), 254-263.

Streib, G. F. (1985). Social stratification and aging. In R. Binstock and E. Shanas (Eds.), *Handbook of aging and the social sciences*, 2nd ed. New York, NY: Van Nostrand Reinhold.

Teague, M. L. (1980). Aging and leisure: A social psychological perspective. In S. E. Iso-Ahola (Ed.), *Social psychological perspectives on leisure and recreation* (pp. 219-260). Springfield, IL: Charles C. Thomas, Publisher.

Teague, M. L., MacNeil, R. D., and Hitzhusen, G. L. (Eds.), (1982). *Perspectives on leisure and aging in a changing society.* Columbia, MO: Department of Recreation and Park Administration.

U.S. Department of Health and Human Services. (1992). *Clinical practice guidelines: Urinary incontinence in adults.* Rockville, MD: Agency for Health Care Policy and Research.

Voelkl, J. E. (1989). "The daily experiences of older adults residing in institutional environments." Unpublished Doctoral Dissertation. University Park, PA: The Pennsylvania State University.

Waters, E. B. and Goodman, J. (1990). *Empowering older adults*. San Francisco, CA: Jossey-Bass Inc, Publishers.

Zborowski, M. (1962). Aging and recreation. *Journal of Gerontology*, *17*, 302-309.

Zimmerman, M. A., Israel, B. A., Schulz, A., and Checkoway, B. (1992). Further explorations in empowerment theory: An empirical analysis of psychological empowerment. *American Journal of Community Psychology*, *20*, 707-727.

Zoerink, D. A. (1988). Effects of short-term leisure education program upon leisure functioning of young people with spina bifida. *Therapeutic Recreation Journal, xxii,* third quarter, 44-52.

Resources

Flaghouse Special Populations
150 N. MacQuesten Parkway
Mount Vernon, NY 10550
(800) 793-7900
(Sensory airflow mat, therabands, weights, massager, bulb hand dynamometer, and other recreation therapy equipment)

Briggs Corporation
P.O. Box 1698
Des Moines, IA 50306-1698
(800) 247-2343
(*MDS forms,* adaptive recreational supplies, and equipment)

Buyer's Guide to Games
B & P Publishing Co.
575 Boylston St.
Boston, MA 02116
(617) 536-5536
(Includes reviews and ratings of games)

Worldwide Games
P.O. Box 517
Colchester, CT 06415-0517
(800) 888-0987
(A variety of gross motor and table games)

Creative Crafts International
16 Plains Rd. Box 819
Essex, CT 06426

Therapy Skill Builders
3839 E. Bellevue, Dept. C
Tucson, Arizona 85716

Wolverine Sports
745 State Circle
Box 1941
Ann Arbor, Michigan 48106

Delta Society and Pet Partners Program
321 Burnett Ave. South
Third Floor
Renton, WA 98055-2569
(206) 226-7357

Horticulture/Gardening Program
Cornell Cooperative Extension
Gardening Department
111 Broadway
New York, NY 10006

National Council for Therapeutic Recreation Certification
P.O. Box 479
Thiells, NY 10984-0479
(914) 947-4346

American Therapeutic Recreation Association
P.O. Box 15215
Hattiesburg, MS 39404-5215
(800) 553-0304

To obtain copies of the *Farrington Assessments* and/or the *Comprehensive Leisure Constraints Assessment,* please contact coauthor Shelley Martin at the following address:

Shelley Martin
145 Arbor Bluff Drive
Pleasant Gap, PA 16823

For questions or further information concerning this text, please contact coauthor Linda Buettner at the following address:

Linda Buettner
Decker School of Nursing
Attention: Linda Buettner
Binghamton University
Binghamton, NY 13902

Appendix A
The Farrington Assessments

The Farrington Therapeutic Recreation Data Sheet

Resident: ______________________ **#:** ____________

Room #: ____________ **DOB:** ____________ **Date:** ____________

Personal Data

Date of Admission: ____________ Social Security #: ____________

Family Contact: ____________ Phone: ____________

Occupation: ____________ Retirement Date: ____________

Name of Spouse or Significant Other: ____________

Names of children: ____________

Religion: ____________ Marital Status: ____________

Education: ____________

Safety

Dietary Restrictions or Problems: ____________

Food/Environmental Allergies: ____________

Check all that apply:

_____ Resident eats independently

_____ Resident smokes

_____ Resident drinks alcohol

_____ Resident wanders or elopes

_____ Resident eats nonfood items

_____ Resident poses a danger to self or others

_____ Resident sensitive to sunlight

Physician's Permission Granted For:

_____ Activities Program _____ Outings _____ Alcohol Consumption

_____ Exposure to Sun _____ Smoking _____ Exercises

Physician's Signature: ____________

Farrington Cognitive Function Assessment

Resident: ______________________________ **#:** ______________

Room #: ________________________ **Month and Year:** ______________

Directions: Place a score in the box for each question asked. Place and X in the box of that question was not asked. Total the score in each column and divide by the number of questions asked for numerical comparisons. 0 = incorrect or no answer; 1 = partially correct answer; 2 = totally correct answer.

Date of assessment:																				
1. Residents first name																				
2. Resident's last name																				
3. Name of facility																				
4. Name of city																				
5. Name of state																				
6. Name of hometown																				
7. Today' weather																				
8. Present time																				
9. Present segment of day (a.m./p.m.)																				
10. Last meal																				
11. Next meal																				
12. Day of week																				
13. Date (21st)																				
14. Month																				
15. Present season																				
16. Last season																				
17. Next season																				
18. Next holiday																				
19. Last holiday																				
20. Present year																				
21. Identify a "pen"																				
22. Name a piece of clothing																				
23. Name a kind of fruit																				
24. Name a color																				
25. Separate objects by color																				
26. Separate objects by shape																				
27. Draw a circle																				
28. Raise your own right hand																				
29. What is 4 + 8?																				
30. How many apples is a dozen?																				
Rate mood: A = Agitated; F = Frustrated; U = Uncooperative; O = OK mood																				
Total Score																				
# of questions asked																				
Adjusted score (total/# of questions)																				

Signature: ______________________________ Date: ______________

The Farrington Initial Therapeutic Recreation Assessment

Resident: ______________________ **#:** __________

Room #: ______________________ **Admission Date:** __________

Age: ______________________ **Assessment Date:** __________

Constraints to Leisure

I. Intrapersonal	II. Interpersonal	III. Structural
COGNITIVE	COMMUNICATION	SITUATIONAL
Not oriented x 3	Speech impairment	Limited financial resources
Not alert	Unable to read or write	Limited time for leisure
Short attention span	Hearing impairment	Decline in health status
Memory impairment	Does not follow directions	
EMOTIONAL	SOCIAL	PHYSICAL
Negative self-esteem	Interacts w/ objects	Impaired mobility
Symptoms of depression	Interacts w/ others 1:1	Needs assistance—mobility
Anxiety	Interacts in small group	Reduced endurance
Anger	Interacts in large group	Unsteady gait
Flat affect	Passive interaction	Impaired range of motion
Fears	Competitive	Paralysis
Easily frustrated	Cooperative	Amputation/Prosthesis
Learned helplessness	Neat appearance	Contractures
Enjoys leading others	Independent mobility	
LOCUS OF CONTROL	FAMILY	SENSORY
Sense of independence	Lacks family	Visual impairment
Sense of helplessness	Lacks significant other	Hearing impairment
Refuses activities	Little family contact	Taste impairment
Difficulty making decisions	Frequent family contact	Smell impairment
Difficulty identifying choices	Family losses and grief	Tactile impairment
LEISURE ATTITUDES	BEHAVIORAL	LEISURE AWARENESS
Does not value leisure	Tics (involuntary mvmnt)	Lacks leisure resources
Does not enjoy leisure	Refuses to respond	Lacks family leis. resources
Unable to identify leisure	Exposes genitals in public	Unaware of leisure activities
Dissatisfied w/ own leisure	Takes clothes off in public	Lacks knowledge of leisure
Unrealistic self-expectations	Screams	Understands rights
SPIRITUAL	Verbally abusive	Desires leisure goals
Participates in religion	Physically aggressive	Aware of assessment
Content w/ own spirituality	Pacing	
Agnostic	Wanders	
Atheistic	Restless	
Fears mortality	Dangerous to self or others	

Signature: ______________________ Date: __________

The Farrington Strengths Assessment

SCORING KEY: 0 = NO; X = YES

Resident: ______________________________ **Assessment Date:** ____________________

PHYSICAL STRENGTHS:

- [ ] Independently mobile
- [ ] Ambulates ad lib
- [ ] Enjoys eating
- [ ] Independent ADLs
- [ ] Endurance
- [ ] Strength
- [ ] Flexibility
- [ ] Range of motion
- [ ] Fine motor skills
- [ ] Gross motor skills
- [ ] Other: ____________

ENVIRONMENTAL/SITUATIONAL STRENGTHS:

- [ ] Financial resources
- [ ] Health status
- [ ] Enjoys leisure activities
- [ ] Adjusting to placement
- [ ] Values leisure
- [ ] Awareness of leisure activities
- [ ] Adequate time for leisure
- [ ] Able to adapt to leisure
- [ ] Other: ____________

SENSORY STRENGTHS:

- [ ] Vision
- [ ] Smell
- [ ] Taste
- [ ] Touch
- [ ] Hearing
- [ ] Other: ____________

COMMUNICATIONS STRENGTHS:

- [ ] Speech
- [ ] Reading
- [ ] Writing
- [ ] Uses a hearing aid
- [ ] Alternative communication
- [ ] English primary
- [ ] Enjoys conversation
- [ ] Initiates conversation
- [ ] Initiates topics

INTERPERSONAL STRENGTHS:

- [ ] Imagination
- [ ] Interaction w/ object
- [ ] Aggregate
- [ ] 1:1 interaction
- [ ] Unilateral
- [ ] Multilateral
- [ ] Cooperation
- [ ] Competition
- [ ] Makes eye contact
- [ ] Uses facial expressions
- [ ] Enjoys social interaction
- [ ] Enjoys small group settings
- [ ] Enjoys large group settings
- [ ] Likes to interact w/ staff
- [ ] Interacts w/ residents
- [ ] Gets along with roommate
- [ ] Assertive
- [ ] Initiates interaction
- [ ] Passive participation
- [ ] Active participation
- [ ] Makes new friends
- [ ] Appearance
- [ ] Family and/or friends
- [ ] Enjoys pets

EMOTIONAL & ATTITUDE STRENGTHS:

- [ ] Able to identify feelings
- [ ] Expressive feelings
- [ ] Able to identify own needs
- [ ] Has motivation
- [ ] Prefers to be active
- [ ] Enjoys new experiences
- [ ] Plans own leisure
- [ ] Internal source of evaluation
- [ ] Positive self-esteem
- [ ] Strong identity
- [ ] Independent
- [ ] Satisfied with own life
- [ ] Spirituality or religion
- [ ] Able to identify choices
- [ ] Able to make choices
- [ ] Internal locus of control
- [ ] Playfulness
- [ ] Enjoys pleasure
- [ ] Shows interest/curiosity
- [ ] Creative
- [ ] Positive attitude
- [ ] Feels competence
- [ ] Feels control
- [ ] Enjoys humor

COGNITIVE STRENGTHS:

- [ ] Enjoys reminiscing
- [ ] Able to identify objects
- [ ] Able to identify colors
- [ ] Able to identify shapes
- [ ] Able to categorize objects
- [ ] Able to recall past events
- [ ] Able to solve math problems
- [ ] Able to follow directions
- [ ] Able to pair objects
- [ ] Able to pair words
- [ ] Knows own name
- [ ] Oriented x 3
- [ ] Able to identify family
- [ ] Able to identify staff
- [ ] Able to locate own room

The Farrington Leisure History

Resident: ______________________ #: __________

Room #: ______________________ Date: __________

Games

- [ ] Billiards
- [ ] Bingo
- [ ] Baseball/Softball
- [ ] Badminton
- [ ] Boxing
- [ ] Bocce Ball
- [ ] Auto Racing
- [ ] Checkers
- [ ] Croquet
- [ ] Chess
- [ ] Cards
- [ ] Board Games
- [ ] Word Finds
- [ ] Crossword Puzzles
- [ ] Gambling
- [ ] Fencing
- [ ] Hockey
- [ ] Horseshoes
- [ ] Quoits
- [ ] Jigsaw Puzzles
- [ ] Pub Games
- [ ] Darts
- [ ] Field Hockey
- [ ] Football
- [ ] Golf
- [ ] Horseracing
- [ ] Karate/Judo/etc.
- [ ] Shuffleboard
- [ ] Squash/Handball
- [ ] Tennis
- [ ] Volleyball
- [ ] Archery
- [ ] Basketball
- [ ] Fitness/Exercise
- [ ] Gymnastics
- [ ] Table Tennis
- [ ] Watching Sports
- [ ] Bowling
- [ ] Miniature Golf
- [ ] Soccer
- [ ] Wrestling

Social

- [ ] Babysitting
- [ ] Club Meetings
- [ ] Parties
- [ ] Religious Org.
- [ ] Shopping
- [ ] Social Drinking
- [ ] Telephoning
- [ ] Volunteering
- [ ] Writing Letters
- [ ] Ham Radio
- [ ] Church
- [ ] Encounter Groups
- [ ] Night Clubs
- [ ] Taverns
- [ ] Pets
- [ ] Church Suppers
- [ ] Dancing
- [ ] Dining Out
- [ ] Fraternal Orgztn
- [ ] Political Activity
- [ ] Civic organizations
- [ ] Family Parties
- [ ] Sitting on Porch
- [ ] Visiting Friends
- [ ] Volunteer Fire Dep't
- [ ] Vol. Ambulance
- [ ] Auctions

Outdoors

- [ ] Driving
- [ ] Boating
- [ ] Flying
- [ ] Gardening
- [ ] Jogging
- [ ] Motorcycling
- [ ] Skindiving
- [ ] Diving
- [ ] Parachuting
- [ ] Surfing
- [ ] Go to the Beach
- [ ] Water Skiing
- [ ] Camping
- [ ] Mountain Climbing
- [ ] Rollerskating
- [ ] Sailing
- [ ] Snowmobiling
- [ ] ATVs/3-wheelers
- [ ] Swimming
- [ ] Walking
- [ ] Hiking
- [ ] Fishing
- [ ] Hunting/Trapping
- [ ] Bird Watching
- [ ] Kite Flying
- [ ] Sunbathing
- [ ] Bicycling
- [ ] Backpacking
- [ ] Canoeing
- [ ] Riding in a Car
- [ ] Horsebackriding
- [ ] Iceskating
- [ ] Nature Walks
- [ ] Parades
- [ ] Picnicking
- [ ] Rec. Vehicles
- [ ] Amusement Parks
- [ ] Skiing
- [ ] Target Shooting
- [ ] Butterfly Watching
- [ ] Rock Climbing

Cultural

- [ ] Acting
- [ ] Carpentry
- [ ] Cooking/Baking
- [ ] Model Building
- [ ] Crafts/Metalwork
- [ ] Design Clothes
- [ ] Electronics
- [ ] Leatherworking
- [ ] Needlework
- [ ] Plays
- [ ] Quilting
- [ ] Museums
- [ ] Auto Repair
- [ ] Antique Cars
- [ ] Ceramics
- [ ] Collecting
- [ ] Crochet
- [ ] Decorating
- [ ] Draw Houseplans
- [ ] Lectures/Educat'n
- [ ] Flower Arranging
- [ ] Meditation
- [ ] Musical Instrument
- [ ] Weaving/Knitting
- [ ] Creative Writing
- [ ] Auto Care
- [ ] Bookbinding
- [ ] Composing Music
- [ ] Poetry
- [ ] Repairs/Remodel
- [ ] Radio/Music
- [ ] Photography
- [ ] Sewing
- [ ] Concerts
- [ ] Traveling
- [ ] Antiques
- [ ] Movies/TV
- [ ] Paint/Draw
- [ ] Pottery/Sculpture
- [ ] Reading
- [ ] Woodworking

The Farrington Current Leisure Interest Profile

Resident: ______________________ **#:** __________

Room #: ______________________ **Date:** __________

Games
- [ ] Billiards
- [ ] Bingo
- [ ] Baseball/Softball
- [ ] Badminton
- [ ] Boxing
- [ ] Bocce Ball
- [ ] Auto Racing
- [ ] Checkers
- [ ] Croquet
- [ ] Chess
- [ ] Cards
- [ ] Board Games
- [ ] Word Finds
- [ ] Crossword Puzzles
- [ ] Gambling
- [ ] Fencing
- [ ] Hockey
- [ ] Horseshoes
- [ ] Quoits
- [ ] Jigsaw Puzzles
- [ ] Pub Games
- [ ] Darts
- [ ] Field Hockey
- [ ] Football
- [ ] Golf
- [ ] Horseracing
- [ ] Karate/Judo/etc.
- [ ] Shuffleboard
- [ ] Squash/Handball
- [ ] Tennis
- [ ] Volleyball
- [ ] Archery
- [ ] Basketball
- [ ] Fitness/Exercise
- [ ] Gymnastics
- [ ] Table Tennis
- [ ] Watching Sports
- [ ] Bowling
- [ ] Miniature Golf
- [ ] Soccer
- [ ] Wrestling

Social
- [ ] Babysitting
- [ ] Club Meetings
- [ ] Parties
- [ ] Religious Org.
- [ ] Shopping
- [ ] Social Drinking
- [ ] Telephoning
- [ ] Volunteering
- [ ] Writing Letters
- [ ] Ham Radio
- [ ] Church
- [ ] Encounter Groups
- [ ] Night Clubs
- [ ] Taverns
- [ ] Pets
- [ ] Church Suppers
- [ ] Dancing
- [ ] Dining Out
- [ ] Fraternal Orgztn
- [ ] Political Activity
- [ ] Civic organizations
- [ ] Family Parties
- [ ] Sitting on Porch
- [ ] Visiting Friends
- [ ] Volunteer Fire Dep't
- [ ] Vol. Ambulance
- [ ] Auctions

Outdoors
- [ ] Driving
- [ ] Boating
- [ ] Flying
- [ ] Gardening
- [ ] Jogging
- [ ] Motorcycling
- [ ] Skindiving
- [ ] Diving
- [ ] Parachuting
- [ ] Surfing
- [ ] Go to the Beach
- [ ] Water Skiing
- [ ] Camping
- [ ] Mountain Climbing
- [ ] Rollerskating
- [ ] Sailing
- [ ] Snowmobiling
- [ ] ATVs/3-wheelers
- [ ] Swimming
- [ ] Walking
- [ ] Hiking
- [ ] Fishing
- [ ] Hunting/Trapping
- [ ] Bird Watching
- [ ] Kite Flying
- [ ] Sunbathing
- [ ] Bicycling
- [ ] Backpacking
- [ ] Canoeing
- [ ] Riding in a Car
- [ ] Horsebackriding
- [ ] Iceskating
- [ ] Nature Walks
- [ ] Parades
- [ ] Picnicking
- [ ] Rec. Vehicles
- [ ] Amusement Parks
- [ ] Skiing
- [ ] Target Shooting
- [ ] Butterfly Watching
- [ ] Rock Climbing

Cultural
- [ ] Acting
- [ ] Carpentry
- [ ] Cooking/Baking
- [ ] Model Building
- [ ] Crafts/Metalwork
- [ ] Design Clothes
- [ ] Electronics
- [ ] Leatherworking
- [ ] Needlework
- [ ] Plays
- [ ] Quilting
- [ ] Museums
- [ ] Auto Repair
- [ ] Antique Cars
- [ ] Ceramics
- [ ] Collecting
- [ ] Crochet
- [ ] Decorating
- [ ] Draw Houseplans
- [ ] Lectures/Educat'n
- [ ] Flower Arranging
- [ ] Meditation
- [ ] Musical Instrument
- [ ] Weaving/Knitting
- [ ] Creative Writing
- [ ] Auto Care
- [ ] Bookbinding
- [ ] Composing Music
- [ ] Poetry
- [ ] Repairs/Remodel
- [ ] Radio/Music
- [ ] Photography
- [ ] Sewing
- [ ] Concerts
- [ ] Traveling
- [ ] Antiques
- [ ] Movies/TV
- [ ] Paint/Draw
- [ ] Pottery/Sculpture
- [ ] Reading
- [ ] Woodworking

Leisure Interests and Needs

Resident Name ______________________

Resident #: ______________

Room #: ______________ Birth Date: ______________ Date: __________

Part I. Leisure Interest Types

Directions: Rate the following types of leisure activities in order of your preference on a scale of 1 to 10.

#1 = Most Preferred #10 = Least Preferred

- ☐ Arts and Crafts
- ☐ Educational
- ☐ Games
- ☐ Outdoors and Nature
- ☐ Sports and Exercise
- ☐ Collecting
- ☐ Cultural, including Art and Music
- ☐ Socializing and Visiting
- ☐ Clubs and Organizations
- ☐ Volunteering

Part II. Leisure Needs

Directions: Rate the following reasons as to their importance in your selection of leisure activities on a scale of 1 to 8.

#1 = Most Important #8 = Least Important

- ☐ Relaxation
- ☐ Excitement
- ☐ Fun
- ☐ Companionship
- ☐ Health
- ☐ Accomplishment
- ☐ Escape
- ☐ Rejuvenation

Resident/Family Signature: ______________________ Date: __________

TR Signature: ______________________ Date: __________

Comprehensive Leisure Constraints Assessment

SCORING KEY: 0 = NO X = YES

Resident: ______________________ **Assessment Date:** ______________

Physical Constraints:

- Impaired mobility
- Uses wheelchair
- Uses cane or walker
- Uses gerichair
- Amputation
- Prosthesis
- Needs assistance w/ mobility
- Unsteady gait
- Needs assistance w/ transfer
- Non-weightbearing
- Paralysis: ____________
- Usually not out of bed
- Contractures
- Independently mobile
- Ambulates: __________
- Difficulty eating: ________
- Needs assistance with eating
- Feeding tube
- Needs to lose weight
- Nausea
- Vertigo or dizziness
- Sleeps during day
- Frequent naps
- Awake at night
- Impaired range of motion
- Impaired fine motor skills
- Impaired gross motor skills
- Reduced endurance
- Tires easily
- Complains of pain
- Incontinence
- Catheter or Colostomy
- Uses oxygen
- Dialysis
- Needs assistance w/ ADLs
- Other: ____________

Environmental/Situational Constraints:

- Limited financial resources
- Decline in health status
- Ecological barriers
- Lacks equipment for activity
- Needs to adjust to placement
- Lacks leisure skills
- Unaware of leisure activities
- Unable to adapt leisure
- Limited time for leisure
- Architectural barriers
- Disturbed by noise
- Other: ____________

Sensory Constraints:

- Vision impairment
- Smell impairment
- Taste impairment
- Tactile impairment
- Hearing impairment
- Other: ____________

Communication Constraints:

- Difficulty speaking
- Unable to read or write
- Difficulty being understood
- Unable to communicate
- Refuses to communicate
- Difficulty hearing
- Uses a hearing aid
- Alternative communication
- Foreign language primary
- English primary
- Converses with others
- Receptive to conversation
- Initiates conversation
- Initiates topics
- Other: ____________

Interpersonal Constraints:

- Difficulty imagining
- Difficulty interacting w/ object
- Difficulty w/ aggregation
- Difficulty w/ 1 : 1 interaction
- Difficulty w/ unilateral
- Difficulty w/ multilateral
- Difficulty w/ cooperation
- Difficulty making eye contact
- Few facial expressions
- Withdrawn
- Refuses social interaction
- Anxiety in group settings
- Dislikes social interaction
- Prefers to interact w/ staff
- Difficult interaction w/ residents
- Refuses contact w/ residents
- Unassertive
- Difficulty initiating interaction
- Passive participation
- Active participation
- Difficulty waiting turn
- Difficulty making new friends
- Poor appearance
- Lacks friends
- Has many friends
- Manipulative
- Enjoys pets

Additional Comments:

Therapeutic Recreation Signature: ______________________ Date: __________

Comprehensive Leisure Constraints Assessment (continued)

Emotional and Attitude Constraints:

- [ ] Flat effect/no expression
- [ ] Unable to identify feelings
- [ ] Unable to express feelings
- [ ] Blanket emotional response
- [ ] Unable to identify own needs
- [ ] Prior psychiatric diagnosis
- [ ] History of abuse
- [ ] History of addiction
- [ ] Present psychiatric diagnosis
- [ ] Taking psychotropic meds
- [ ] Does not enjoy activities
- [ ] Lacks motivation
- [ ] Prefers to do nothing
- [ ] Reduced activity level
- [ ] Refuses activity participation
- [ ] Resists new experiences
- [ ] Refuses to plan on leisure
- [ ] Does not value leisure
- [ ] Does not enjoy leisure

- [ ] Low self esteem
- [ ] Lacks own identity
- [ ] Dependent on others
- [ ] Lacks confidence in abilities
- [ ] Feelings of worthlessness
- [ ] Dissatisfied with own life
- [ ] Lacks spirituality or religion
- [ ] Questions meaning of life
- [ ] Anxiety about leaving room
- [ ] Anxious/nervous/panic
- [ ] Feelings of fear
- [ ] Feelings of paranoia
- [ ] Hallucinations
- [ ] Difficulty identifying choices
- [ ] Feels little choice
- [ ] Difficulty making choices
- [ ] External locus of control
- [ ] Feelings of helplessness
- [ ] External source of evaluation

- [ ] Feelings of guilt
- [ ] Multiple losses/recent grief
- [ ] Feels sad
- [ ] Cries
- [ ] Feels tired much of the time
- [ ] Frequently irritable
- [ ] Feels angry
- [ ] Outbursts of rage
- [ ] Lack of pleasure
- [ ] Lack of interest (apathetic)
- [ ] Feels discontented frequently
- [ ] Frequent complaints
- [ ] Negative outlook
- [ ] Difficulty being playful
- [ ] Lacks feelings of competence
- [ ] Lacks feelings of control
- [ ] Dissatisfied w/ own leisure
- [ ] Unrealistic self expectations
- [ ] Other: ____________

Cognitive Status:

- [ ] Unresponsive to stimulus
- [ ] Unable to identify objects
- [ ] Unable to identify colors
- [ ] Unable to identify shapes
- [ ] Unable to categorize objects
- [ ] Unable to recall recent events
- [ ] Unable to recall past events
- [ ] Unable to solve math probs
- [ ] Unable to follow directions
- [ ] Unable to pair objects
- [ ] Unable to pair words
- [ ] Memory problem
- [ ] Responds appropriately

- [ ] Repetitive speech
- [ ] Repetitive motion
- [ ] Rambling/incoherent speech
- [ ] Uses nonsense words
- [ ] Smiles inappropriately
- [ ] Laughs inappropriately
- [ ] Short attention span
- [ ] Confused
- [ ] Unable to focus attention
- [ ] Difficulty understanding
- [ ] Not oriented x 3
- [ ] Enjoys reminiscing about past
- [ ] Unable to copy patterns

- [ ] Unable to state own name
- [ ] Not responsive to own name
- [ ] Unable to identify family
- [ ] Unable to identify TR staff
- [ ] Unable to locate own room
- [ ] Unable to locate activities
- [ ] Recent change in medication
- [ ] Recent change in room, etc.
- [ ] Recent hospitalization
- [ ] Recent infection
- [ ] Recent fall/head injury
- [ ] Sudden change in cognition
- [ ] Other: ____________

Family Interaction:

- [ ] Does not have family
- [ ] Family at a distance
- [ ] Little or no family contact
- [ ] Res. desires more autonomy

- [ ] Family is controlling
- [ ] Family is argumentative
- [ ] Family has frequent c/o
- [ ] Difficult family interaction

- [ ] Has few family members
- [ ] Recent family loss/grief (2yr)
- [ ] Family does not share leisure
- [ ] Other: ____________

Behavior Problems:

- [ ] Involuntary movements
- [ ] Inappropriate body exposure
- [ ] Physically abusive to self
- [ ] Physically combative
- [ ] Trespasses
- [ ] Repeated questions/phrases
- [ ] Noisy/Disruptive

- [ ] Demanding staff
- [ ] Argumentative
- [ ] Aggressive
- [ ] Easily agitated
- [ ] Impatient
- [ ] Easily frustrated
- [ ] Refuses care or meds

- [ ] Refuses to respond
- [ ] Verbally abusive
- [ ] Paces/Restless
- [ ] Wanders/Elopes
- [ ] Dangerous to self or others
- [ ] Takes others things
- [ ] Other: ____________

Therapeutic Recreation Signature: ______________________ Date: __________

Comprehensive Therapeutic Recreation Assessment Summary

Resident: ______________________ **#:** ____________

Room #: __________ **Date:** ______________

Summary of Functioning Levels

Physical: ______________________

Mental: ______________________

Emotional: ______________________

Social: ______________________

Financial: ______________________

Spiritual: ______________________

Occupational: ______________________

LEISURE

Control: ______________________

Competence: ______________________

Attitudes: ______________________

Playfulness: ______________________

Participation: ______________________

Needs:

- ☐ Relaxation
- ☐ Companionship
- ☐ Escape
- ☐ Health
- ☐ Accomplishment
- ☐ Rejuvenation
- ☐ Excitement
- ☐ Fun

Leisure Interests

Major Past Interests: ______________________

Major Current Interests: ______________________

Comparision of Past and Present and Types: ______________________

Comprehensive Therapeutic Recreation Assessment Summary (continued)

Leisure Constraints

Intraindividual Constraints

Physical: ______________________________

Environmental: ______________________________

Sensory: ______________________________

Extraindividual Constraints

Communication: ______________________________

Interpersonal: ______________________________

Family: ______________________________

Behavioral: ______________________________

Interindividual Constraints

Emotional: ______________________________

Attitudes: ______________________________

Cognative: ______________________________

Needs

Physical: ______________________________

Safety and Trust: ______________________________

Love and Belonging: ______________________________

Strengths	Weaknesses

TR Signature: ______________________________ Date: __________

Resident/Family Signature: ______________________________ Date: __________

The Farrington Therapeutic Recreation Plan of Care

Resident: ______________________ #: __________

Room #: __________ DOB: ______________ Date: __________

Problem/Needs List	Strengths List
1.	1.
2.	2.
3.	3.
4.	4.
5.	5.

Care Plan

Goal	Performance Measure	Objectives/Intervention

Therapeutic Interventions Recommended:

- [ ] Newcomer Group
- [ ] Remotivation
- [ ] Sensory Stimulation
- [ ] Guided Imagery
- [ ] Horticulture Therapy
- [ ] Art Therapy
- [ ] Leisure Education
- [ ] Reminiscing
- [ ] Assertiveness Training
- [ ] Hug Therapy
- [ ] Grief Group
- [ ] Reality Orientation
- [ ] Relaxation
- [ ] Pet Therapy
- [ ] Music Therapy
- [ ] Validation
- [ ] Values Clarification
- [ ] Empowerment
- [ ] Resocialization
- [ ] Humor

Signature: ______________________ Date: __________

Appendix B
Overall Therapeutic Recreation Programming Guidelines

Therapeutic Recreation Programming Guidelines

I. Recreation therapy programs should be planned to:

a. Show an awareness of resident's needs and interests;
b. Have the resident's care plan objectives included;
c. Plan for a structured activity;
d. Have an alternative activity planned;
e. Secure the proper resources in advance; and
f. Make sure the activity area is safe.

II. Recreation therapists need to be aware and knowledgeable of the residents in their programs.

a. Know the names of the residents and their special needs.
b. Understand the best form of communication to use with each resident in the program.
c. Be aware of the resident's strengths, interests, and motivations.

III. Programs being conducted must meet resident needs.

a. Residents should be involved in the program.
b. Staff should be actively involved.
c. Staff should be sensitive to resident's likes and dislikes.
d. Flexibility—modify approaches should be implemented if needed.

IV. Choose appropriate activities to achieve treatment objectives.

a. Build trust and a sense of security into the program.
b. Allow for choice making and self-expression.
c. Provide mental and physical stimulation.
d. Promote social growth and opportunities for socialization.
e. Build in feedback for the resident.

V. Use creativity in planning and implementing programs.

a. Take advantage of natural surroundings.
b. Employ talents of specialists.
c. Use different types of music or themes to reach residents.

Appendix C
Sample Recreation Therapy Flow Chart

Rating Scale for Recreation Therapy

Resident: ______________________ **Group:** ______________

BEHAVIOR SEEN	DATE:	No	At Times	Often	100%
Comes to group willingly					
Makes eye contact					
Is alert and awake throughout					
Responds to verbal prompting					
Makes appropriate responses					
Connects group material with personal experience					
Makes leisure preferences known					
Performs movement actions					
Stays total time					
Appears calm and relaxed at closure					

Any agitation behavior (repetitious mannerisms, pick, grab, or throw things, yells, aggressive or inappropriate behaviors):

Goals:

Comments:

Therapist: ______________________

Appendix D
Therapeutic Recreation Protocols for Residents with Dementia

Suggested Programs

Recreation

1. Leisure Lounge
2. Raingutter Bocce League—Other adapted sports
3. Special Events
4. Gardening
5. Kitchen Activities—Make Your Own Snacks—Setting the Table
6. Computer Games/Table Games
7. Community Outings
8. Hobbies of Choice

Leisure Education

1. Build Your Own Games
2. Special Event Preparation Group
3. Newsletter Group
4. Sensory Cooking/Herb Gardening/Tea Time Social Club
5. Photography Group

Recreation Therapy to Improve Function

1. Art Therapy Program
2. Hands and Feet Stim Program
3. Cognitive Therapy Group
4. Sensory Air Mat Therapy
5. Stim Box Therapy
6. Falls Prevention Program
   a. Walking Program
   b. Exercise for Function

Daily Program Schedule for Residents with Dementia

Morning Routine

6:00-8:00	Morning wake-up—Toileting and dressing for breakfast
7:00-8:00	Early Risers Walking Group
8:00-9:00	Dining room—BREAKFAST
9:00-10:00	Finishing Touches Program (e.g., morning care, shaving, cleaning glasses, checking, hearing aids, make-up and jewelry)
10:00-10:30	M–F Exercise for function group
10:30	Nutrition cart
10:40-11:40	M–F Air mat therapy
11:40-12:00	Dining room sensory game/cognitive activity and prepare for lunch
12:00-1:00	LUNCH

Afternoon Routine

1:00-2:00	Rest time in room or leisure lounge
2:00-2:15	Wake-up and toileting
2:15-2:45	Make your own snack program—Blender cooking
3:00-4:00	Therapeutic Recreation
	M: Photography Club
	T: Community Garden Club
	W: Bibliotherapy Program—Poems, reading, writing.
	TH: Art Therapy Program
	F: Animal Assisted Therapy or Kids
	SAT: Table games/adapted bingo
	SUN: Family tea and activities
4:00-5:00	Cognitive Therapy: "Price is Right"
5:00	DINNER

Evening Routine

6:00-6:30	Local news and views (Orientation)
6:30	Toileting and wash-up time
	Leisure lounge open
7:00	Small group activities, family visits, visits with kids, animals, walks outside
8:00-9:30	Hydration—Ready for bed—Sleepy-time music

Programs for Residents with Dementia

Leisure Lounge

The philosophy of the Leisure Lounge is based on the Leisure Education and Recreation Participation segments of the Leisurability Model (Peterson & Gunn, 1984). The concept of normalization is an important one in this program. Older adults in the community have an eclectic set of interests and activities in which they participate. Senior centers in our communities flourish when based on this concept; quality and variety are vital. The Leisure Lounge idea promotes the same variety and quality for persons with dementia. It allows older adults with cognitive impairments time to socialize, engage in simple activities of their choosing, engage in shared activities, find their own stimulation, or simply to watch others. It is an alternative to providing structured programming in all the possible time slots of the day.

GOAL: The goal of the Leisure Lounge is to provide an environment for free choice, socialization, and activity.

OBJECTIVES:

1. Encourage residents to move around and initiate activity.
2. Facilitate age appropriate social interactions.
3. Empower residents.
4. Allow residents to provide themselves with appropriate stimulation or retreat time.
5. Reduce problematic behaviors.

The Leisure Lounge will be staffed by one or more staff and should be open in one or two hour time slots every day. For example, from 1:30 to 3:00 and 6:30 to 8:00. It will include gross motor games, arts and crafts, letter writing, refreshments, and individual attention. Residents can wander in and out, touch, interact, or retreat to a cozy chair according to the individual's desires.

Falls Prevention Program

The falls prevention program was established to reduce the number of falls in older adults with dementia. It has three parts, and is interdisciplinary. Part I is the morning walking group. In this program identified residents are assisted in graded walking activities. The distances are individualized to match the residents' endurance levels and ambulation abilities. Distances are charted on a weekly basis and increased as residents improve. The walking program ends with the residents at the dining area, ready for breakfast. Part II of the program is geriatric exercise. This program is presented three times weekly. Strength, coordination, and flexibility activities are provided and residents are assisted in step by step movements. Part III is the sensory integration group.

Entrance Criteria: Two falls in a given month or a single fall in two consecutive months.

Exit Criteria: No falls for three months.

PART I—EARLY RISERS WALKING PROGRAM

Goal: To increase lower extremity strength and overall endurance.

Objectives:

1. To increase the scope and duration of activities that can be performed at or below a safe heart range.
2. To maintain or improve ambulation skills.
3. To reduce early morning falls at wake up time by providing a meaningful, structured therapeutic activity.

Day: M–F

Time: 7:00 to 7:30 a.m.

Group size: 7 to 10 residents will be individually provided with the program.

Staff: Recreation therapist, physical therapy assistant, nursing staff.

Methodology: A group of 7 to 10 residents will be selected for the early risers walking program. Therapy staff will assist residents in walking or wheeling their own chairs a prescribed distance based on assessment of endurance and overall health. Blood pressures and heart rates will be periodically monitored during and after the activity. The distance of the walk will increase as the residents' abilities improve.

Selection Criteria: Resident demonstrates unsteady gait, need to improve or maintain cardiovascular endurance.

Exit Criteria: Ability to walk 20 minutes without tiring; three months without falling.

Support needs: Residents are awake, dressed, and wearing good shoes for walking. Adequate staff for number of residents in program.

Monitoring: Incident reports for falls.

PART II—EXERCISE FOR FUNCTION

Goals: To improve or prevent regression of levels of health. To maintain or improve overall flexibility and strength for daily living skills and maximum independence.

Time: Monday–Wednesday–Friday 10:00-10:30

Group size: 7 to 10 residents with individualized assistance for each task.

Staff: Therapist and assistant

Methodology: The residents will be surveyed for musical likes and dislikes. The exercise program will be choreographed with the music the group selects. The following movements/exercises will be included in each session:

Activities for Range of Motion:

a. Head rotation and flexion
b. Shoulder shrug
c. Back stretch: Sit up straight, bend forward, sit up straight
d. Knee lifts
e. Leg extension
f. Arm extension: Palms together, slide arms outward, back inward and then upward
g. Hand extension

Activities for Strength:

a. Elastic or theraband activities
b. Free hand weights or water jug passing
c. Chair push-ups
d. Gross motor games

Activities for Endurance:

a. Walking to and from the program
b. Exerpedic system or exercise bike
c. Gross motor games

Selection Criteria: Residents showing functional losses due to weakness, loss of endurance, or flexibility.

Exit Criteria: Residents show independence in basic ADLs.

Support Needs: two or three staff per 10 residents, therabands or elastic, dowels, weights, balls, balloons, and assorted games.

Monitoring: Strength, overall flexibility, endurance testing every 10 weeks. Overall functioning will be tested using the Timed Manual Performance Instrument (TMP) every three months.

PART III—SENSORY AIR MAT THERAPY PROGRAM

The sensory air mat program is a safe and therapeutically proven method for promoting mobility and relaxation responses in residents who are physically frail and behaviorally difficult. It is also appropriate for residents who have poor balance, are immobile, or unable to seek sensory stimulation.

Goals: The activities on the air mat fall into several specific goal areas with the ultimate purpose of improving total body movement and functioning of the individual:

1. To improve one-to-one communication and appropriate responses.
2. To improve developmental movements which lay the foundation for ADLs.
3. To improve body awareness and aid in understanding ones' relative position in space.
4. To improve balance while engaging in recreational activities.
5. To improve transfer and ambulation skills which lead to independence in seeking recreational activities.
6. To promote free movement and empowerment.
7. To provide a guided relaxation experience.

Precautions: Consideration must be given to general safety precautions as well as those incurred in therapeutic procedures such as tone increase in irregular and hypertonic muscles, sensory overload, over inhibition, and seizure precaution. Its influence on the autonomic nervous system may be recognized by flushing, blanching, perspiring, nausea, or yawning. These signs are indicators that the amount of stimulation should be reduced.

Selection Criteria: Resident displays loss of strength, flexibility, balance, ability to relax, balance, or ambulation skills.

Exit Criteria: Resident displays safe, independent mobility and the ability to relax.

Support needs: Two staff and one air mat per session.

Monitoring: Residents are tested every ten weeks for strength, flexibility, and ambulation. Overall agitation levels will be assessed by nursing service personnel. Falls and mobility will be assessed through incident report and physical therapy evaluations.

For Successful Programming

1. Simplicity and consistency.
2. Provide choices, but structure the options—empower the resident.
3. Be ready with a step-by-step breakdown.
4. Inclusion—Residents with dementia need a full program of activities.
5. Include recreation, leisure education and therapy.
6. Improve communication.
7. Supervise, but don't take over.
8. Adapt your programs to meet the needs of the residents.
9. Small groups are best with one-to-one attention within the group.
10. Normalize your programs.
11. Be prepared to offer a diversion.
12. Program to maximize independence—IMPROVE STRENGTH, FLEXIBILITY, and ENDURANCE.

Art Therapy/Build Your Own Games

Service: New dementia unit

Day/Time:

Location: Activity room

Goals: To provide each resident with an opportunity to express herself through art; to improve or maintain upper extremity function; to improve coordination between eye and hand; to take part in activities that are meaningful and useful.

Methodology: All tasks will be planned to match the functional levels of the residents involved. The process of completing each activity is what is considered most important; not the final product. Large pieces will be used with close therapeutic supervision to promote success experiences in each session. Self-expression will be encouraged in each project. The types of projects include:

1. Making large posters and wall hangings for the unit.
2. Mosaic type projects using texture.
3. Painting rocks and other large objects.
4. Sponge and template art.
5. Gluing and painting game pieces for leisure lounge.
6. Mask making and sculpture.
7. Group theme projects like—"If I were stranded on an island I would want..."

Entrance criteria: Past interest in art/crafts and communication or upper extremity use difficulties. Inability to structure own leisure.

Exit criteria: Improved communication or upper extremity function and ability to structure own leisure.

Sensory Cooking Program

Service: New dementia unit

Day/time:

Location: Activity room

Staff: Recreation therapist/certified occupational therapy assistant/nursing staff

Goals: Residents will improve or maintain the ability to follow one-step directions. Residents will improve or maintain the ability to talk about favorite foods/recipes from the past. Residents will improve or maintain the ability to open, stir, pour, and serve foods. Residents will use adaptive cooking equipment to complete simple tasks. Residents will wash hands before and after cooking group without becoming agitated. Residents will make simple choices regarding foods and tasks presented in the cooking program. Residents will eat using appropriate dining etiquette.

Methodology: Tasks like opening, cutting, and stirring will be assigned to various members of the group based on ability levels. Self mobility skills will also be reinforced by asking residents to walk or wheel to and from the program and help to attain necessary objects for the group. Dementia often affects the residents' appetite in a negative way. This program will focus on the smells and textures most appealing to residents in the mid- to later-stages of Alzheimer's. Comparisons will be made between fresh, canned, and frozen foods. Special interests of the residents' will be used in the planning process.

Entrance criteria: Resident is losing interest in eating or the ability to follow one-step directions. Resident enjoyed cooking/eating out in the past. Resident expresses an interest in the program.

Exit criteria: Resident is no longer having eating problems. Resident can complete one-step tasks. Residents' interests change. Resident has attained goal.

Photography Group

Service: Dementia Unit

Day/Time:

Location: Outdoors during good weather. Around the unit in poor weather.

Staff: Recreation therapist/occupational therapist/nursing staff

Goals: Residents will improve or maintain the ability to make simple choices. Residents will identify topics of interest to photograph. Residents will share equipment with others in the group. Residents will demonstrate the ability to take a clear photo. Residents will arrange pictures or slides for others to view. Residents will share the pictures or slides with others. Residents will take part in small group interactions as evidenced by talking to another resident or staff member in each session.

Methodology: A small group of residents who express an interest in photography will learn to take 35mm (slides and prints) and Polaroid pictures. The group will select the themes, the area, and the equipment to be used in each session. The residents will take turns shooting the photos. The group will create displays for the unit and scrapbooks of the various themes. Members of the group will also be encouraged to photograph the special events that take place at the facility. A monthly slide or video show will be presented for the community to view.

Entrance criteria: Expresses interest in photography. Is able to hold the camera. Needs to work on following one-step directions, group interactions, or making simple choices.

Exit criteria: Is no longer interested in photography. Attains goals.

Requirements: Cameras, film, staff, scrapbooks, slide projector.

Raingutter Bocce League

Service: Dementia unit

Day/Time: Tuesday–Thursday evenings 6:30

Location: Outdoor activity area

Staff: Therapist and aide

Goals: Residents will maintain or improve the ability to reach, grasp, and release a bocce size ball. Residents will demonstrate the ability to follow one-step directions, take turns, and cheer for each other appropriately. Residents will interact with one peer and staff coach in each session. Residents will make simple choices (e.g., color of ball, place in the line-up) in each session. Residents will have fun and enjoy the activity.

Methodology: Residents will be assessed for the ability to roll a bocce size ball a distance of 15 to 20 feet. The residents will make a large colorful target area with a point system for scoring. Residents will use a six foot plastic raingutter if needed to assist them in rolling the balls. After a few practice sessions teams will be formed and unit staff will serve as coaches. The league games will be scheduled during the evenings.

Entrance criteria: Interest in the program. Unoccupied leisure time in the evening. Needs to maintain or improve direction following, upper extremity function, and social skills.

Exit criteria: No longer interested in program. Is able to structure own leisure. Attains goals.

Price Is Right—Cognitive group

Service: Dementia unit

Day/Time: Weekdays 4:00 to 5:00

Location: Dining room

Staff: Recreation therapist and speech therapist

Equipment/Materials: Empty food boxes with prices hidden.

Goals: Residents will maintain or improve cognitive skills as evidenced by the ability to make a choice between two objects, converse on a topic, and understand money/pricing of food. Residents will make a choice between two objects six times per session. Residents will verbally select a price when asked "how much do you think this costs." Residents will discuss products that look familiar at least one time per session. Residents will interact verbally in a small group by contributing to the conversation about the product.

Methodology: Many residents are lethargic and have behavior problems in the late afternoon time frame. In addition, many residents are unmotivated to attend the evening meal. This program is designed around familiar food products to stimulate appetite, cognitive skills, and conversation. This program is structured for residents who are in the moderate to later stages of Alzheimer's disease. Two boxes or cartons will be held up and a question will be asked of the group. Then each resident in the program will be asked individually "which product costs more" (or less). Another version of this uses a 4 x 6 inch card with the price on it. Residents are asked which carton goes with the price. At the end of each question the right answer will be given and the residents will have the opportunity to talk about the products. For example: "I just showed you a box of rice crispies and corn flakes. What is your favorite breakfast cereal?"

Entrance criteria: Cognitive impairment, loss of communication skills, poor appetite, interest in the program.

Exit criteria: Able to make simple choices, follow directions, carry on a simple conversation. Has adequate appetite. No longer interested in program.

Music Therapy

Service: New dementia unit

Day/Time: Tuesday, Thursday, Friday 9:30-10:30 a.m.

Group size: 10 to 15 residents with individualized assistance for each task.

Staff: Music therapist and assistant

Goals: To provide each resident with an opportunity to (1) express herself through music, (2) to make choices, (3) initiate responses, (4) stimulate memory recall, (5) maintain or improve range of motion, (6) improve eye-hand coordination, (7) encourage verbal expression, and (8) to reduce agitation.

Methodology: The residents will be assessed for past/present music interests. Program will start with a hello song and close with a good-bye song. Activities during the session will include: activities for eye-hand coordination, activities for range of motion, activities for using slow familiar songs to encourage memory recall, verbal expression, relaxation.

Selection criteria: Past/current interest in music, periods of agitation, loss of flexibility or coordination.

Exit criteria: No longer interested and has met treatment goals.

Newsletter Group

Service: New dementia unit

Day/Time: Wednesday at 2:00

Location: Outdoors and indoors

Goals: To provide the participants the opportunity to talk about issues (now and from times past), work together in a small group setting, type or work with a computer, copy machine, and deliver the finished product to other residents and staff.

Methodology: Residents (3 to 5) will select the columns to be included from a list of options such as: Health Tips, Sports & Leisure, Upcoming Events, Recipes, Talk of the Season. Residents will be encouraged to talk about the topics and notes will be taken. One or two residents will assist with typing. Another one or two will assist with copying the letter and delivery. One finished newsletter will come out each month.

Entrance criteria: Able to verbalize thoughts, needs to improve socialization or contact with other residents, enjoys reading, is interested.

Exit criteria: Attained goals, no longer interested in newsletter group.

See sample newsletter (next page)

A Leisurely Look

July 21, 1995

Staff: Viola, Loraine, Vivenne, Florence and Linda

Health Tip: How to avoid falling—

- Look where you are going.
- Use the handrails in the hallways.
- If there is something on the floor pick it up so no one slips.
- Always where a good fitting shoe.
- Keep your legs strong...walking is good exercise.

Favorite Modes of Transportation

Loraine and Viola agree that wheelchairs and cars are not very good ways to get around.

Viola always preferred a bicycle when she was younger. It was cheap and didn't pollute the air.

Florence enjoyed riding her horse to the store and just for pleasure. She rode bareback most of the time.

Vivienne argued that she would take a ride in a convertible anytime!!

Every Friday in August we will be having the chance to make our own pancakes for breakfast!

Three go to hospital

This week three of our friends went to Tompkins hospital. Myrtle was treated for a broken hip. Doris had a bout with pneumonia. Eva was treated and has returned to our unit. We hope they all feel better soon.

The Good Old Summer Time

It has been very hot this summer. We have a walk through porch but it is very sunny out there. Bring a hat or sunglasses if you plan to sit out.

The month of August has the theme "Good Old Summer Time." All of the activities and special events will focus on this theme.

We will be making homemade lemonade every Wednesday morning. Stop by for a **FREE** glass. Be sure to wear your shorts for an extra surprise!

Things we like to do in the summer:

- swimming
- picnics
- sitting under a tree
- drinking ice cold lemonade or iced tea
- going on walks in the evening

Look for more news next month!

Appendix E

Quality Assurance Sample Documents

Clinical Activity: Recreation therapy progress notes

Indicators:

a. Recreation therapy progress notes will be written in a timely fashion.
b. Recreation therapy progress notes will include all pertinent information.

Criteria:

a. Timeliness
    (1) New admissions will receive 30 day notes for the next six months.
    (2) Residents will receive 90 day notes thereafter.
b. Pertinent information
    (1) See attached note writing guidelines to assure:
        - notes are written to the care plan,
        - notes are programmatically descriptive,
        - notes are behaviorally descriptive.

Monitoring:

a. Timeliness
    (1) 90 percent threshold for evaluation of timeliness is considered acceptable.
    (2) Retrospective chart review of 3 to 5 notes per unit every quarter by QA director for recreation.
b. Pertinent information
    (1) 85 percent threshold for evaluation is considered acceptable.
    (2) Retrospective chart review completed quarterly.
    (3) By the QA Director for recreation therapy.

Note Writing Guidelines:

a. Notes are to be written to the care plan goal.
   (1) State the goal you are working on in the note.
   (2) Clear, concise information about progress toward the goal should be included.
b. Describe the recreation therapy programming the resident received (not just attendance but participation).
   (1) The recreation therapy activities the resident attended should be entered in the body of the note.
   (2) Careful documentation of the actual participation of the resident.
c. Describe the behavior of the resident in the recreation therapy setting.
   (1) If the resident was difficult to manage in the program it should be documented in the body of the note.
   (2) Positive and negative behaviors should be related to content of the recreation program. Indicate the trigger for the negative or inappropriate behaviors seen.
   (3) Indicate if the resident was alert, calm, active or passive, verbal or able to make choices known, able to walk or wheel to program, and the resident's level of socialization.
d. Progress and future directions for recreation therapy.
   (1) Did the resident progress, maintain, or regress in regard to his or her treatment goal?
   (2) Does the change seen indicate a revision in the care plan is needed.
   (3) List recommendations for the future.

Progress Note Quality Assurance Checklist

Was the note:

YES NO

___ ___ 1. Completed on or before the 30 (90) day requirement.

Were the following items included in the progress note:

YES NO

___ ___ 1. The goal being worked on was highlighted or mentioned,
___ ___ 2. Name the specific programs the resident attended,
___ ___ 3. The length of time in each program the resident was active,
___ ___ 4. What active things the resident did,
___ ___ 5. Did the resident initiate any activities,
___ ___ 6. What passive things the resident did,
___ ___ 7. Was the resident alert or confused,
___ ___ 8. Did the resident verbalize or make choices known,
___ ___ 9. Did the resident interact socially with peers or staff,
___ ___ 10. Level of socialization,
___ ___ 11. Was the resident calm during and at the end of the program,
___ ___ 12. If not calm, what specific behaviors were seen and what triggered the behavior,
___ ___ 13. Did the resident independently walk or wheel to and from the program—what distance was covered,
___ ___ 14. Attainment or progress toward goals, and
___ ___ 15. Future treatment recommendations or revisions needed.

QA Director completing the monitoring:

____

Date of monitoring: __________________

Monitor for (name of therapist):

____

Clinical Activity: Recreation Therapy Assessments

Indicator: Assessments will include all pertinent information.

Criteria:

a. Threshold for acceptable evaluation is 90 percent.
b. Adhere to guidelines for recreation therapy assessment to assess:
   (1) Current skills, talents, aptitudes, cultural, spiritual, and recreational interests.
   (2) Past skills, talents, aptitudes, cultural, spiritual, and recreational interests.
   (3) Constraints to recreation/leisure.
   (4) Problems, strengths, motivations, and treatment recommendations.

Monitoring:

a. Retrospective chart review of three to five assessments per unit.
b. Completed quarterly.
c. By QA Director for recreation therapy.

Clinical Activity: Treatment Planning

Indicator: Recreation therapy goals/objectives for care plans will be written in a timely fashion.

Criteria:

a. Recreation therapy objective on assessment will be selected in compliance with assessment standards:
   (1) Initial assessment—seven days.
   (2) Transfer assessments—thirty days.
   (3) Annual assessments—each year.

b. Recreation therapy objective will be reflected in the care plan.

Monitoring:

a. Retrospective chart review of 3 to 5 charts per unit.
b. Completed quarterly.
c. By the QA director for recreation therapy.

Clinical Activity: Resident Satisfaction

Indicator: Residents will be satisfied with recreation therapy staff and activities available in the facility.

Criteria:

a. Resident and/or advocate will answer positively on at least 75 percent of items from:
   (1) Recreation Satisfaction Form.
   (2) Therapist Effectiveness Form.

b. New programs will be developed to meet residents' interests.
   (1) Suggestion box
   (2) Resident Council Meetings

Method:

a.
   (1) Satisfaction forms will be provided to residents and/or advocates for the residents during each recreation program offering in each unit of the facility.
   (2) Therapist/recreation staff effectiveness forms will be provided to residents and/or family advocates during each recreation program offering in each unit of the facility.

b.
   (1) Each unit will have a suggestion box for recreational activities. New activities will be introduced on every unit quarterly based on the suggestions.
   (2) Resident council will identify activities they would like to see provided during the next quarter.

Monitoring:

(1) Satisfaction forms will be distributed and tabulated quarterly.
(2) Suggestion box responses will be collected, documented, and passed on to appropriate staff to address the need or interest.
(3) Minutes from resident council meetings will identify interest areas for recreational programs.
(4) QA director for recreation/activity therapy will ensure satisfaction levels are met.

Resident Satisfaction Survey

Activity: ______________________ Therapist: ______________

Date: ______________________ Unit: ______________

Did you enjoy this activity?	YES	NO
Have you done this before?	YES	NO
Would you like to do this again?	YES	NO

RATE THE ACTIVITY ON A SCALE OF 1 TO 5:

1	2	3	4	5
(Great)	(Very Good)	(Good)	(Just OK)	(Not Very Good)

What would you rather do during leisure time?

Signed: ______________________________ Date: __________

Therapist Effectiveness Survey

Therapist's Name: ______________________

1.	My therapist was interested in me:	YES	NO
2.	Therapist kept the activity interesting:	YES	NO
3.	Therapist was usually on time:	YES	NO
4.	Therapist took an active part:	YES	NO
5.	Therapist cared about me:	YES	NO
6.	Therapist helped me feel better:	YES	NO
7.	Therapist talked to me:	YES	NO
8.	Therapist was courteous:	YES	NO
9.	Therapist was knowledgeable:	YES	NO
10.	Therapist showed respect for me:	YES	NO
11.	Therapist won my trust:	YES	NO
12.	Therapist was sensitive to my needs:	YES	NO

Rate The Therapist

1	2	3	4
Outstanding	Very Effective	Effective	Needs Improvement

Signed: ______________________________ Date: ________________

Clinical Activity: Recreation Therapy Programs

Indicator: Programs will be need and outcome based

Criteria:

a. Uses the Recreation Therapy Program Guidelines.
b. 90 percent threshold of acceptance for evaluation.

Monitoring:

a. Direct observation of ongoing therapeutic recreation programs.
b. On each unit in the facility.
c. By the QA Director for recreation therapy.
d. On a quarterly basis.

Appendix F
The Minimum Data Set (MDS) Forms—Version 2.0

MINIMUM DATA SET (MDS) — *VERSION 2.0*

FOR NURSING HOME RESIDENT ASSESSMENT AND CARE SCREENING

BASIC ASSESSMENT TRACKING FORM

SECTION AA. IDENTIFICATION INFORMATION

1.	RESIDENT NAME ⊛	a. (First) b. (Middle Initial) c. (Last) d. (Jr./Sr.)
2.	GENDER ⊛	1. Male 2. Female
3.	BIRTHDATE ⊛	Month – Day – Year
4.	RACE/ ⊛ ETHNICITY	1. American Indian/Alaskan Native 2. Asian/Pacific Islander 3. Black, not of Hispanic origin 4. Hispanic 5. White, not of Hispanic origin
5.	SOCIAL ⊛ SECURITY AND ⊛ MEDICARE NUMBERS [C in 1st box if non Med. no.]	a. Social Security Number b. Medicare number (or comparable railroad insurance number)
6.	FACILITY PROVIDER NO. ⊛	a. State No. b. Federal No.
7.	MEDICAID NO. *["+" if pending, "N" if not a Medicaid recipient]* ⊛	
8.	REASONS FOR ASSESS-MENT	[Note—Other codes do not to this form] a. Primary reason for assessment 1. Admission assessment (required by day 14) 2. Annual assessment 3. Significant change in status assessment 4. Significant correction of prior assessment 5. Quarterly review assessment 0. *NONE OF ABOVE* b. ***Special codes for use with supplemental assessment types in Case Mix demonstration states or other states where required*** *1. 5 day assessment* *2. 30 day assessment* *3. 60 day assessment* *4. Quarterly assessment using full MDS form* *5. Readmission/return assessment* *6. Other state required assessment*
9.	SIGNATURES OF PERSONS COMPLETING THESE ITEMS:	

a. Signatures	Title	Date
b.		Date

GENERAL INSTRUCTIONS

Complete this information for submission with all full and quarterly assessments (Admission, Annual, Significant Change, State or Medicare required assessments, or Quarterly Reviews, etc.).

⊛ = Key items for computerized resident tracking

☐ = When box blank, must enter number or letter

[a.] = When letter in box, check if condition applies

Code "—" if information unavailable or unknown

TRIGGER LEGEND

1 - Delirium
2 - Cognitive Loss/Dementia
3 - Visual Function
4 - Communication
5A - ADL-Rehabilitation
5B - ADL-Maintenance
6 - Urinary Incontinence and Indwelling Catheter
7 - Psychosocial Well-Being
8 - Mood State
9 - Behavioral Symptoms
10A - Activities (Revise)
10B - Activities (Review)
11 - Falls
12 - Nutritional Status
13 - Feeding Tubes
14 - Dehydration/Fluid Maintenance
15 - Dental Care
16 - Pressure Ulcers
17 - Psychotropic Drug Use
18 - Physical Restraints

1 of 8

MDS 2.0 10/18/94N

MINIMUM DATA SET (MDS) — *VERSION 2.0*

FOR NURSING HOME RESIDENT ASSESSMENT AND CARE SCREENING

BACKGROUND (FACE SHEET) INFORMATION AT ADMISSION

SECTION AB. DEMOGRAPHIC INFORMATION

1.	DATE OF ENTRY	*Date the stay began. Note — Does not include readmission if record was closed at time of temporary discharge to hospital, etc. In such cases, use prior admission date.* ☐☐–☐☐–☐☐☐☐ Month Day Year
2.	ADMITTED FROM (AT ENTRY)	1. Private home/apt. with no home health services 2. Private home/apt. with home health services 3. Board and care/assisted living/group home 4. Nursing home 5. Acute care hospital 6. Psychiatric hospital, MR/DD facility 7. Rehabilitation hospital 8. Other
3.	LIVED ALONE (PRIOR TO ENTRY)	0. No 1. Yes 2. In other facility
4.	ZIP CODE OF PRIOR PRIMARY RESIDENCE	☐☐☐☐☐
5.	RESIDENTIAL HISTORY 5 YEARS PRIOR TO ENTRY	*(Check all settings resident lived in during 5 years prior to date of entry given in item AB1 above.)* Prior stay at this nursing home a. Stay in other nursing home b. Other residential facility — board and care home, assisted living, group home c. MH/psychiatric setting d. MR/DD setting e. *NONE OF ABOVE* f.
6.	LIFETIME OCCUPATION(S) (Put "/" between two occupations)	
7.	EDUCATION (*Highest level completed*)	1. No schooling 5. Technical or trade school 2. 8th grade/less 6. Some college 3. 9-11 grades 7. Bachelor's degree 4. High school 8. Graduate degree
8.	LANGUAGE	*(Code for correct response)* a. Primary Language 0. English 1. Spanish 2. French 3. Other b. If other, specify
9.	MENTAL HEALTH HISTORY	Does resident's RECORD indicate any history of mental retardation, mental illness, or developmental disability problem? 0. No 1. Yes
10.	CONDITIONS RELATED TO MR/DD STATUS	*(Check all conditions that are related to MR/DD status that were manifested before age 22, and are likely to continue indefinitely)* Not applicable — no MR/DD (Skip to AB11) a. MR/DD with organic condition Down's syndrome b. Autism c. Epilepsy d. Other organic condition related to MR/DD e. MR/DD with no organic condition f.
11.	DATE BACKGROUND INFORMATION COMPLETED	☐☐–☐☐–☐☐☐☐ Month Day Year

☐ = When box blank, must enter number or letter

a. = When letter in box, check if condition applies

Code "—" if information unavailable or unknown

SECTION AC. CUSTOMARY ROUTINE

1.	CUSTOMARY ROUTINE (*In year prior to DATE OF ENTRY to this nursing home, or year last in community if now being admitted from another nursing home*)	***(Check all that apply. If all information UNKNOWN, check last box only.)***
		CYCLE OF DAILY EVENTS
		Stays up late at night (e.g., after 9 pm) a.
		Naps regularly during day (at least 1 hour) b.
		Goes out 1+ days a week c.
		Stays busy with hobbies, reading, or fixed daily routine d.
		Spends most of time alone or watching TV e.
		Moves independently indoors (with appliances, if used) f.
		Use of tobacco products at least daily g.
		NONE OF ABOVE h.
		EATING PATTERNS
		Distinct food preferences i.
		Eats between meals all or most days j.
		Use of alcoholic beverage(s) at least weekly k.
		NONE OF ABOVE l.
		ADL PATTERNS
		In bedclothes much of day m.
		Wakens to toilet all or most nights n.
		Has irregular bowel movement pattern o.
		Showers for bathing p.
		Bathing in PM q.
		NONE OF ABOVE r.
		INVOLVEMENT PATTERNS
		Daily contact with relatives/close friends s.
		Usually attends church, temple, synagogue (etc.) t.
		Finds strength in faith u.
		Daily animal companion/presence v.
		Involved in group activities w.
		NONE OF ABOVE x.
		UNKNOWN — Resident/family unable to provide information y.

END

SECTION AD. FACE SHEET SIGNATURES

SIGNATURES OF PERSONS COMPLETING FACE SHEET:

a. Signature of RN Assessment Coordinator			Date
b. Signatures	Title	Sections	Date
c.			Date
d.			Date
e.			Date
f.			Date
g.			Date

NOTE: Normally, the MDS Face Sheet is completed once, when an individual first enters the facility. However, the face sheet is also required if the person is reentering this facility after a discharge where return had not previously been expected. It is not completed following temporary discharges to hospitals or after therapeutic leaves/home visits.

MINIMUM DATA SET (MDS) — *VERSION 2.0*
FOR NURSING HOME RESIDENT ASSESSMENT AND CARE SCREENING
FULL ASSESSMENT FORM
(Status in last 7 days, unless other time frame indicated)

SECTION A. IDENTIFICATION AND BACKGROUND INFORMATION

1.	RESIDENT NAME	a. (First) b. (Middle Initial) c. (Last) d. (Jr./Sr.)
2.	ROOM NUMBER	
3.	ASSESSMENT REFERENCE DATE	a. *Last day of MDS observation period* Month — Day — Year b. Original (0) or corrected copy of form (enter number of correction)
4a.	DATE OF REENTRY	Date of reentry from most recent temporary discharge to a hospital in last 90 days (or since last assessment or admission if less than 90 days) Month — Day — Year
5.	MARITAL STATUS	1. Never married 2. Married 3. Widowed 4. Separated 5. Divorced
6.	MEDICAL RECORD NO.	
7.	CURRENT PAYMENT SOURCES FOR N.H. STAY	*(Billing Office to indicate; check all that apply in last 30 days)* Medicaid per diem a. Medicare per diem b. Medicare ancillary part A c. Medicare ancillary part B d. CHAMPUS per diem e. VA per diem f. Self or family pays for full per diem g. Medicaid resident liability or Medicare co-payment h. Private insurance per diem (including co-payment) i. Other per diem j.
8.	REASONS FOR ASSESSMENT [*Note—If this is a discharge or reentry assessment, only a limited subset of MDS items need be completed*]	a. Primary reason for assessment 1. Admission assessment (required by day 14) 2. Annual assessment 3. Significant change in status assessment 4. Significant correction of prior assessment 5. Quarterly review assessment 6. Discharged—return not anticipated 7. Discharged—return anticipated 8. Discharged prior to completing initial assessment 9. Reentry 0. NONE OF ABOVE b. *Special codes for use with supplemental assessment types in Case Mix demonstration states or other states where required* 1. 5 day assessment 2. 30 day assessment 3. 60 day assessment 4. Quarterly assessment using full MDS form 5. Readmission/return assessment 6. Other state required assessment
9.	RESPONSIBILITY/ LEGAL GUARDIAN	*(Check all that apply)* Legal guardian a. Other legal oversight b. Durable power of attorney/health care c. Durable power of attorney/ financial d. Family member responsible e. Patient responsible for self f. *NONE OF ABOVE* g.
10.	ADVANCED DIRECTIVES	*(For those items with supporting documentation in the medical record, check all that apply)* Living will a. Do not resuscitate b. Do not hospitalize c. Organ donation d. Autopsy request e. Feeding restrictions f. Medication restrictions g. Other treatment restrictions h. *NONE OF ABOVE* i.

SECTION B. COGNITIVE PATTERNS

1.	COMATOSE	*(Persistent vegetative state/no discernible consciousness)* 0. No 1. Yes *(If yes, skip to Section G)*
2.	MEMORY	*(Recall of what was learned or known)* a. Short-term memory OK—seems/appears to recall after 5 minutes 0. Memory OK 1. Memory problem **2** b. Long-term memory OK—seems/appears to recall long past 0. Memory OK 1. Memory problem **2**
3.	MEMORY/ RECALL ABILITY	*(Check all that resident was normally able to recall during last 7 days)* Current season a. Location of own room b. Staff names/faces c. That he/she is in a nursing home d. *NONE OF ABOVE are recalled* e.
4.	COGNITIVE SKILLS FOR DAILY DECISION-MAKING	*(Made decisions regarding tasks of daily life)* 0. *INDEPENDENT*—decisions consistent/reasonable 1. *MODIFIED INDEPENDENCE*—some difficulty in new situations only **2** 2. *MODERATELY IMPAIRED*—decisions poor; cues/ supervision required **2** 3. *SEVERELY IMPAIRED*—never/rarely made decisions **2, 5B**
5.	INDICATORS OF DELIRIUM—PERIODIC DISORDERED THINKING/ AWARENESS	*(Code for behavior in the last 7 days.)* [*Note: Accurate assessment requires conversations with staff and family who have direct knowledge of resident's behavior over this time.*] 0. Behavior not present 1. Behavior present, not of recent onset 2. Behavior present, over last 7 days appears different from resident's usual functioning (e.g., new onset or worsening) a. EASILY DISTRACTED—(e.g., difficulty paying attention; gets sidetracked) **1, 17*** b. PERIODS OF ALTERED PERCEPTION OR AWARENESS OF SURROUNDINGS—(e.g., moves lips or talks to someone not present; believes he/she is somewhere else; confuses night and day) **1, 17*** c. EPISODES OF DISORGANIZED SPEECH—(e.g., speech is incoherent, nonsensical, irrelevant, or rambling from subject to subject; loses train of thought) **1, 17*** d. PERIODS OF RESTLESSNESS—(e.g., fidgeting or picking at skin, clothing, napkins, etc.; frequent position changes; repetitive physical movements or calling out) **1, 17*** e. PERIODS OF LETHARGY—(e.g., sluggishness; staring into space; difficult to arouse; little body movement) **1, 17*** f. MENTAL FUNCTION VARIES OVER THE COURSE OF THE DAY—(e.g., sometimes better, sometimes worse; behaviors sometimes present, sometimes not) **1, 17***
6.	CHANGE IN COGNITIVE STATUS	Resident's cognitive status, skills, or abilities have changed as compared to status of 90 days ago (or since assessment if less than 90 days) 0. No change 1. Improved 2. Deteriorated **1, 17***

SECTION C. COMMUNICATION/HEARING PATTERNS

1.	HEARING	*(With hearing appliance, if used)* 0. *HEARS ADEQUATELY*—normal talk, TV, phone 1. *MINIMAL DIFFICULTY* when not in quiet setting **4** 2. *HEARS IN SPECIAL SITUATIONS ONLY*—speaker has to adjust tonal quality and speak distinctly **4** 3. *HIGHLY IMPAIRED*/absence of useful hearing **4**
2.	COMMUNICATION DEVICES/ TECHNIQUES	*(Check all that apply during last 7 days)* Hearing aid, present and used a. Hearing aid, present and not used regularly b. Other receptive comm. techniques used (e.g., lip reading) c. *NONE OF ABOVE* d.
3.	MODES OF EXPRESSION	*(Check all used by resident to make needs known)* Speech a. Writing messages to express or clarify needs b. American sign language or Braille c. Signs/gestures/sounds d. Communication board e. Other f. *NONE OF ABOVE* g.
4.	MAKING SELF UNDERSTOOD	*(Expressing information content—however able)* 0. *UNDERSTOOD* 1. *USUALLY UNDERSTOOD*—difficulty finding words or finishing thoughts **4** 2. *SOMETIMES UNDERSTOOD*—ability is limited to making concrete requests **4** 3. *RARELY/NEVER UNDERSTOOD* **4**
5.	SPEECH CLARITY	*(Code for speech in the last 7 days)* 0. *CLEAR SPEECH*—distinct, intelligible words 1. *UNCLEAR SPEECH*—slurred, mumbled words 2. *NO SPEECH*—absence of spoken words
6.	ABILITY TO UNDERSTAND OTHERS	*(Understanding verbal information content—however able)* 0. *UNDERSTANDS* 1. *USUALLY UNDERSTANDS*—may miss some part/ intent of message **2, 4** 2. *SOMETIMES UNDERSTANDS*—responds adequately to simple, direct communication **2, 4** 3. *RARELY/NEVER UNDERSTANDS* **2, 4**
7.	CHANGE IN COMMUNICATION/ HEARING	Resident's ability to express, understand, or hear information has changed as compared to status of *90 days ago* *(or since last assessment if less than 90 days)* 0. No change 1. Improved 2. Deteriorated **17***

☐ = When box blank, must enter number or letter.

[a.] = When letter in box, check if condition applies

Code "—" if information unavailable or unknown

TRIGGER LEGEND
1 - Delirium
2 - Cognitive Loss/Dementia
4 - Communication
5B - ADL Maintenance
17* - Psychotropic Drugs
(For this to trigger, O4a, b, or c must = 1-7)

Resident ________

SECTION D. VISION PATTERNS

1.	VISION	*(Ability to see in adequate light and with glasses if used)* 0. *ADEQUATE*—sees fine detail, including regular print in newspapers/books 1. *IMPAIRED*—sees large print, but not regular print in newspapers/books **3** 2. *MODERATELY IMPAIRED*—limited vision; not able to see newspaper headlines, but can identify objects **3** 3. *HIGHLY IMPAIRED*—object identification in question, but eyes appear to follow objects **3** 4. *SEVERELY IMPAIRED*—no vision or sees only light, colors, or shapes; eyes do not appear to follow objects	
2.	VISUAL LIMITATIONS/ DIFFICULTIES	Side vision problems—decreased peripheral vision (e.g., leaves food on one side of tray, difficulty traveling, bumps into people and objects, misjudges placement of chair when seating self) **3**	a.
		Experiences any of following: sees halos or rings around lights; sees flashes of light; sees "curtains" over eyes	b.
		NONE OF ABOVE	c.
3.	VISUAL APPLIANCES	Glasses; contact lenses; magnifying glass 0. No 1. Yes	

SECTION E. MOOD AND BEHAVIOR PATTERNS

1.	INDICATORS OF DEPRES-SION, ANXIETY, SAD MOOD	***(Code for indicators observed in last 30 days, irrespective of the assumed cause)*** 0. Indicator not exhibited in last 30 days 1. Indicator of this type exhibited up to five days a week 2. Indicator of this type exhibited daily or almost daily (6, 7 days a week)

VERBAL EXPRESSIONS OF DISTRESS

a. Resident made negative statements—e.g., "*Nothing matters; Would rather be dead; What's the use; Regrets having lived so long; Let me die*" 1 or 2 = **8**

b. Repetitive questions—e.g., "*Where do I go; What do I do?*" 1 or 2 = **8**

c. Repetitive verbalizations— e.g., calling out for help ("*God help me*") 1 or 2 = **8**

d. Persistent anger with self or others—e.g., easily annoyed, anger at placement in nursing home; anger at care received 1 or 2 = **8**

e. Self deprecation—e.g., "*I am nothing; I am of no use to anyone*" 1 or 2 = **8**

f. Expressions of what appear to be unrealistic fears—e.g., fear of being abandoned, left alone, being with others 1 or 2 = **8**

g. Recurrent statements that something terrible is about to happen—e.g., believes he or she is about to die, have a heart attack 1 or 2 = **8**

h. Repetitive health complaints—e.g., persistently seeks medical attention, obsessive concern with body functions 1 or 2 = **8**

i. Repetitive anxious complaints/concerns (non-health related) e.g., persistently seeks attention/reassurance regarding schedules, meals, laundry/clothing, relationship issues 1 or 2 = **8**

SLEEP-CYCLE ISSUES

j. Unpleasant mood in morning 1 or 2 = **8**

k. Insomnia/change in usual sleep pattern 1 or 2 = **8**

SAD, APATHETIC, ANXIOUS APPEARANCE

l. Sad, pained, worried facial expressions—e.g., furrowed brows 1 or 2 = **8**

m. Crying, tearfulness 1 or 2 = **8**

n. Repetitive physical movements—e.g., pacing, hand wringing, restlessness, fidgeting, picking 1 or 2 = **8, 17***

LOSS OF INTEREST

o. Withdrawal from activities of interest—e.g., no interest in longstanding activities or being with family/friends 1 or 2 = **7, 8**

p. Reduced social interaction 1 or 2 = **8**

2.	MOOD PERSIS-TENCE	**One or more indicators of depressed, sad or anxious mood were not easily altered by attempts to "cheer up", console, or reassure the resident over last 7 days** 0. No mood indicators 1. Indicators present, easily altered **8** 2. Indicators present, not easily altered **8**
3.	CHANGE IN MOOD	Resident's mood status has changed as compared to status of **90 days ago** (or since last assessment if **less than 90 days**) 0. No change 1. Improved 2. Deteriorated **1, 17***
4.	BEHAVIORAL SYMPTOMS	***(A) Behavioral symptom frequency in last 7 days*** 0. Behavior not exhibited in last 7 days 1. Behavior of this type occurred 1 to 3 days in last 7 days 2. Behavior of this type occurred 4 to 6 days, but less than daily 3. Behavior of this type occurred daily ***(B) Behavioral symptom alterability in last 7 days*** 0. Behavior not present OR behavior was easily altered 1. Behavior was not easily altered

	(A)	(B)
a. WANDERING (moved with no rational purpose, seemingly oblivious to needs or safety) A = 1, 2, or 3 = **9, 11**		
b. VERBALLY ABUSIVE BEHAVIORAL SYMPTOMS (others were threatened, screamed at, cursed at) A = 1, 2, or 3 = **9**		
c. PHYSICALLY ABUSIVE BEHAVIORAL SYMPTOMS (others were hit, shoved, scratched, sexually abused) A = 1, 2, or 3 = **9**		
d. SOCIALLY INAPPROPRIATE/DISRUPTIVE BEHAVIORAL SYMPTOMS (made disruptive sounds, noisiness, screaming, self-abusive acts, sexual behavior or disrobing in public, smeared/threw food/feces, hoarding, rummaged through others' belongings) A = 1, 2, or 3 = **9**		
e. RESISTS CARE (resisted taking medications/injections, ADL assistance, or eating)		

Numeric Identifier ________

5.	CHANGE IN BEHAVIORAL SYMPTOMS	Resident's behavior status has changed as compared to **status of 90 days ago** (or since last assessment if less than 90 days) 0. No change 1. Improved **9** 2. Deteriorated **1, 17***

SECTION F. PSYCHOSOCIAL WELL-BEING

1.	SENSE OF INITIATIVE/ INVOLVE-MENT	At ease interacting with others	a.
		At ease doing planned or structured activities	b.
		At ease doing self-initiated activities	c.
		Establishes own goals **7**	d.
		Pursues involvement in life of facility (e.g., makes/keeps friends; involved in group activities; responds positively to new activities; assists at religious services)	e.
		Accepts invitations into most group activities	f.
		NONE OF ABOVE	g.
2.	UNSETTLED RELATION-SHIPS	Covert/open conflict with or repeated criticism of staff **7**	a.
		Unhappy with roommate **7**	b.
		Unhappy with residents other than roommate **7**	c.
		Openly expresses conflict/anger with family/friends **7**	d.
		Absence of personal contact with family/friends	e.
		Recent loss of close family member/friend	f.
		Does not adjust easily to change in routines	g.
		NONE OF ABOVE	h.
3.	PAST ROLES	Strong identification with past roles and life status **7**	a.
		Expresses sadness/anger/empty feeling over lost roles/status **7**	b.
		Resident perceives that daily routine (customary routine, activities) is very different from prior pattern in the community **7**	c.
		NONE OF ABOVE	d.

SECTION G. PHYSICAL FUNCTIONING AND STRUCTURAL PROBLEMS

1\. (A) ADL SELF-PERFORMANCE—***(Code for resident's PERFORMANCE OVER ALL SHIFTS during last 7 days—Not including setup)***

0. *INDEPENDENT*—No help or oversight—OR—Help/oversight provided only 1 or 2 times during last 7 days
1. *SUPERVISION*—Oversight, encouragement or cueing provided 3 or more times during last 7 days—OR—Supervision (3 or more times) plus physical assistance provided only 1 or 2 times during last 7 days
2. *LIMITED ASSISTANCE*—Resident highly involved in activity; received physical help in guided maneuvering of limbs or other nonweight bearing assistance 3 or more times—OR—More help provided only 1 or 2 times during last 7 days
3. *EXTENSIVE ASSISTANCE*—While resident performed part of activity, over last 7-day period, help of following type(s) provided 3 or more times:
   —Weight-bearing support
   —Full staff performance during part (but not all) of last 7 days
4. *TOTAL DEPENDENCE*—Full staff performance of activity during entire 7 days
8. *ACTIVITY DID NOT OCCUR* during entire 7 days

(B) ADL SUPPORT PROVIDED—***(Code for MOST SUPPORT PROVIDED OVER ALL SHIFTS during last 7 days; code regardless of*** *resident's self-performance classification)*

0. No setup or physical help from staff
1. Setup help only
2. One person physical assist
3. Two+ persons physical assist
8. ADL activity itself did not occur during entire 7 days

			(A) SELF-PERF	(B) SUPPORT
a.	BED MOBILITY	How resident moves to and from lying position, turns side to side, and positions body while in bed A = 1 = **5A**; A = 2, 3, or 4 = **5A, 16**; A = 8 = **16**		
b.	TRANSFER	How resident moves between surfaces—to/from: bed, chair, wheelchair, standing position (EXCLUDE to/from bath/toilet) A = 1, 2, 3, or 4 = **5A**		
c.	WALK IN ROOM	How resident walks between locations in his/her room A = 1, 2, 3, or 4 = **5A**		
d.	WALK IN CORRIDOR	How resident walks in corridor on unit A = 1, 2, 3, or 4 = **5A**		
e.	LOCOMO-TION ON UNIT	How resident moves between locations in his/her room and adjacent corridor on same floor. If in wheelchair, self-sufficiency once in chair A = 1, 2, 3, or 4 = **5A**		
f.	LOCOMO-TION OFF UNIT	How resident moves to and returns from off unit locations (e.g., areas set aside for dining, activities, or treatments). If facility has only one floor, how resident moves to and from distant areas on the floor. If in wheelchair, self-sufficiency once in chair A = 1, 2, 3, or 4 = **5A**		
g.	DRESSING	How resident puts on, fastens, and takes off all items of street clothing, including donning/removing prosthesis A = 1, 2, 3, or 4 = **5A**		
h.	EATING	How resident eats and drinks (regardless of skill). Includes intake of nourishment by other means (e.g., tube feeding, total parenteral nutrition) A = 1, 2, 3, or 4 = **5A**		
i.	TOILET USE	How resident uses the toilet room (or commode, bedpan, urinal); transfers on/off toilet, cleanses, changes pad, manages ostomy or catheter, adjusts clothes A = 1, 2, 3, or 4 = **5A**		
j.	PERSONAL HYGIENE	How resident maintains personal hygiene, including combing hair, brushing teeth, shaving, applying makeup, washing/drying face, hands, and perineum (EXCLUDE baths and showers) A = 1, 2, 3, or 4 = **5A**		

TRIGGER LEGEND
1 - Delirium
3 - Visual Function
5A - ADL Rehabilitation
7 - Psychosocial Well-Being
8 - Mood State
9 - Behavior Symptoms
11 - Falls
17* - Psychotropic Drugs
(*For this to trigger, O4a, b, or c must = 1-7)

Form 39728L MDS 2.0 10/18/94N

Resident ____________________ Numeric Identifier ____________________

2.	**BATHING**	How resident takes full-body bath/shower, sponge bath, and transfers in/out of tub/shower (EXCLUDE washing of back and hair). ***Code for most dependent** in self-performance and support.* A = 1, 2, 3 or 4 = **5A** (A) BATHING SELF-PERFORMANCE codes appear below. (A) (B) 0. Independent—No help provided 1. Supervision—Oversight help only 2. Physical help limited to transfer only 3. Physical help in part of bathing activity 4. Total dependence 8. Activity itself did not occur during entire 7 days *(Bathing support codes are as defined in **Item 1, code B above**)*
3.	**TEST FOR BALANCE** (See training manual)	*(Code for ability during test in the last 7 days)* 0. Maintained position as required in test 1. Unsteady, but able to rebalance self without physical support 2. Partial physical support during test; or stands (sits) but does not follow directions for test 3. Not able to attempt test without physical help a. Balance while standing b. Balance while sitting—position, trunk control 1, 2, or 3 = **17***
4.	**FUNCTIONAL LIMITATION IN RANGE OF MOTION** (see training manual)	*(Code for limitations during **last 7 days** that interfered with daily functions or placed resident at risk of injury)* *(A) RANGE OF MOTION* — 0. No limitation; 1. Limitation on one side; 2. Limitation on both sides *(B) VOLUNTARY MOVEMENT* — 0. No loss; 1. Partial loss; 2. Full loss (A) (B) a. Neck b. Arm—Including shoulder or elbow c. Hand—Including wrist or fingers d. Leg—Including hip or knee e. Foot—Including ankle or toes f. Other limitation or loss
5.	**MODES OF LOCOMOTION**	***(Check all that apply during last 7 days)*** Cane/walker/crutch a. Wheeled self b. Other person wheeled c. Wheelchair primary mode of locomotion d. *NONE OF ABOVE* e.
6.	**MODES OF TRANSFER**	***(Check all that apply during last 7 days)*** Bedfast all or most of time **16** a. Bed rails used for bed mobility or transfer b. Lifted manually c. Lifted mechanically d. Transfer aid (e.g., slide board, trapeze, cane, walker, brace) e. *NONE OF ABOVE* f.
7.	**TASK SEGMENTATION**	Some or all of ADL activities were broken into subtasks during **last 7 days** so that resident could perform them 0. No 1. Yes
8.	**ADL FUNCTIONAL REHABILITATION POTENTIAL**	Resident believes he/she is capable of increased independence in at least some ADLs **5A** a. Direct care staff believe resident is capable of increased independence in at least some ADLs **5A** b. Resident able to perform tasks/activity but is very slow c. Difference in ADL Self-Performance or ADL Support, comparing mornings to evenings d. *NONE OF ABOVE* e.
9.	**CHANGE IN ADL FUNCTION**	Resident's ADL self-performance status has changed as compared to status of **90 days ago** (or since last assessment if less than 90 days) 0. No change 1. Improved 2. Deteriorated

SECTION H. CONTINENCE IN LAST 14 DAYS

1.		CONTINENCE SELF-CONTROL CATEGORIES ***(Code for resident's PERFORMANCE OVER ALL SHIFTS)*** 0. *CONTINENT*—Complete control *(includes use of indwelling urinary catheter or ostomy device that does not leak urine or stool)* 1. *USUALLY CONTINENT*—BLADDER, incontinent episodes once a week or less; BOWEL, less than weekly 2. *OCCASIONALLY INCONTINENT*—BLADDER, 2 or more times a week but not daily; BOWEL, once a week 3. *FREQUENTLY INCONTINENT*—BLADDER, tended to be incontinent daily, but some control present (e.g., on day shift); BOWEL, 2-3 times a week 4. *INCONTINENT*—Had inadequate control. BLADDER, multiple daily episodes; BOWEL, all (or almost all) of the time
a.	**BOWEL CONTINENCE**	Control of bowel movement, with appliance or bowel continence programs, if employed 1, 2, 3 or 4 = **16**
b.	**BLADDER CONTINENCE**	Control of urinary bladder function (if dribbles, volume insufficient to soak through underpants), with appliances (e.g., foley) or continence programs, if employed 2, 3 or 4 = **6**
2.	**BOWEL ELIMINATION PATTERN**	Bowel elimination pattern regular—at least one movement every three days a. Constipation **17*** b. Diarrhea c. Fecal impaction **17*** d. *NONE OF ABOVE* e.
3.	**APPLIANCES AND PROGRAMS**	Any scheduled toileting plan a. Bladder retraining program b. External (condom) catheter **6** c. Indwelling catheter **6** d. Intermittent catheter **6** e. Did not use toilet room/commode/urinal f. Pads/briefs used **6** g. Enemas/irrigation h. Ostomy present i. *NONE OF ABOVE* j.
4.	**CHANGE IN URINARY CONTINENCE**	Resident's urinary continence has changed as compared to status of **90 days ago** (or since last assessment if less than 90 days) 0. No change 1. Improved 2. Deteriorated

SECTION I. DISEASE DIAGNOSES

Check only those diseases that have a relationship to current ADL status, cognitive status, mood and behavior status, medical treatments, nursing monitoring, or risk of death. (Do not list inactive diagnoses)

1. **DISEASES** ***(If none apply, CHECK the NONE OF ABOVE box)***

ENDOCRINE/METABOLIC/ NUTRITIONAL		Hemiplegia/Hemiparesis	v.
Diabetes mellitus	a.	Multiple sclerosis	w.
Hyperthyroidism	b.	Paraplegia	x.
Hypothyroidism	c.	Parkinson's disease	y.
HEART/CIRCULATION		Quadriplegia	z.
Arteriosclerotic heart disease (ASHD)	d.	Seizure disorder	aa.
Cardiac dysrhythmias	e.	Transient ischemic attack (TIA)	bb.
Congestive heart failure	f.	Traumatic brain injury	cc.
Deep vein thrombosis	g.	**PSYCHIATRIC/MOOD**	
Hypertension	h.	Anxiety disorder	dd.
Hypotension **17***	i.	Depression **17***	ee.
Peripheral vascular disease **16**	j.	Manic depression (bipolar disease)	ff.
Other cardiovascular disease	k.	Schizophrenia	gg.
MUSCULOSKELETAL		**PULMONARY**	
Arthritis	l.	Asthma	hh.
Hip fracture	m.	Emphysema/COPD	ii.
Missing limb (e.g., amputation)	n.	**SENSORY**	
Osteoporosis	o.	Cataracts **3**	jj.
Pathological bone fracture	p.	Diabetic retinopathy	kk.
NEUROLOGICAL		Glaucoma **3**	ll.
Alzheimer's disease	q.	Macular degeneration	mm.
Aphasia	r.	**OTHER**	
Cerebral palsy	s.	Allergies	nn.
Cerebrovascular accident (stroke)	t.	Anemia	oo.
Dementia other than Alzheimer's disease	u.	Cancer	pp.
		Renal failure	qq.
		NONE OF ABOVE	rr.

2. **INFECTIONS** ***(If none apply, CHECK the NONE OF ABOVE box)***

Antibiotic resistant infection (e.g., Methicillin resistant staph)	a.	Septicemia	g.
Clostridium difficile (c. diff.)	b.	Sexually transmitted diseases	h.
Conjunctivitis	c.	Tuberculosis	i.
HIV infection	d.	Urinary tract infection in last 30 days **14**	j.
Pneumonia	e.	Viral hepatitis	k.
Respiratory infection	f.	Wound infection	l.
		NONE OF ABOVE	m.

3. **OTHER CURRENT OR MORE DETAILED DIAGNOSES AND ICD-9 CODES**

Dehydration 276.5 = **14**

a. ____________________ •
b. ____________________ •
c. ____________________ •
d. ____________________ •
e. ____________________ •

SECTION J. HEALTH CONDITIONS

1. **PROBLEM CONDITIONS** *(Check all problems present in **last 7 days** unless other time frame is indicated)*

INDICATORS OF FLUID STATUS		Dizziness/Vertigo **11, 17***	f.
Weight gain or loss of 3 or more pounds within a 7 day period **14**	a.	Edema	g.
Inability to lie flat due to shortness of breath	b.	Fever **14**	h.
Dehydrated; output exceeds input **14**	c.	Hallucinations **17***	i.
Insufficient fluid; did NOT consume all/almost all liquids provided during last 3 days **14**	d.	Internal bleeding **14**	j.
OTHER		Recurrent lung aspirations in last 90 days **17***	k.
Delusions	e.	Shortness of breath	l.
		Syncope (fainting) **17***	m.
		Unsteady gait **17***	n.
		Vomiting	o.
		NONE OF ABOVE	p.

TRIGGER LEGEND
3 - Visual Function
5A - ADL Rehabilitation
6 - Urinary Incontinence/Indwelling Catheter
11 - Falls
14 - Dehydration/Fluid Maintenance
16 - Pressure Ulcers
17* - Psychotropic Drugs
(*For this to trigger, O4a, b, or c must = 1-7)

5 of 8

MDS 2.0 10/18/94N

Resident ______ Numeric Identifier ______

2.	PAIN SYMPTOMS	*(Code the highest level of pain present in the last 7 days)* a. FREQUENCY with which resident complains or shows evidence of pain: 0. No pain *(skip to J4)*; 1. Pain less than daily; 2. Pain daily. b. INTENSITY of pain: 1. Mild pain; 2. Moderate pain; 3. Times when pain is horrible or excruciating
3.	PAIN SITE	*(If pain present, check all sites that apply in last 7 days)* Back pain a.; Bone pain b.; Chest pain while doing usual activities c.; Headache d.; Hip pain e.; Incisional pain f.; Joint pain (other than hip) g.; Soft tissue pain (e.g., lesion, muscle) h.; Stomach pain i.; Other j.
4.	ACCIDENTS	*(Check all that apply)* Fell in past 30 days 11, 17* a.; Fell in past 31-180 days 11, 17* b.; Hip fracture in last 180 days 17* c.; Other fracture in last 180 days d.; *NONE OF ABOVE* e.
5.	STABILITY OF CONDITIONS	Conditions/diseases make resident's cognitive, ADL, mood or behavior patterns unstable—(fluctuating, precarious, or deteriorating) a.; Resident experiencing an acute episode or a flare-up of a recurrent or chronic problem b.; End-stage disease, 6 or fewer months to live c.; *NONE OF ABOVE* d.

SECTION K. ORAL/NUTRITIONAL STATUS

1.	ORAL PROBLEMS	Chewing problem a.; Swallowing problem 17* b.; Mouth pain 15 c.; *NONE OF ABOVE* d.
2.	HEIGHT AND WEIGHT	*Record (a.) height in inches and (b.) weight in pounds. Base weight on most recent measure in last 30 days; measure weight consistently in accord with standard facility practice—e.g., in a.m. after voiding, before meal, with shoes off, and in nightclothes.* a. HT (in.) b. WT (lb.)
3.	WEIGHT CHANGE	a. Weight loss—5% or more in last 30 days; or 10% or more in last 180 days 0. No 1. Yes 12; b. Weight gain—5% or more in last 30 days; or 10% or more in last 180 days 0. No 1. Yes
4.	NUTRITIONAL PROBLEMS	Complains about the taste of many foods 12 a.; Regular or repetitive complaints of hunger b.; Leaves 25% or more of food uneaten at most meals 12 c.; *NONE OF ABOVE* d.
5.	NUTRITIONAL APPROACHES	*(Check all that apply in last 7 days)* Parenteral/IV 12, 14 a.; Feeding tube 13, 14 b.; Mechanically altered diet 12 c.; Syringe (oral feeding) 12 d.; Therapeutic diet 12 e.; Dietary supplement between meals f.; Plate guard, stabilized built-up utensil, etc. g.; On a planned weight change program h.; *NONE OF ABOVE* i.
6.	PARENTERAL OR ENTERAL INTAKE	*(Skip to Section L if neither 5a nor 5b is checked)* a. Code the proportion of total calories the resident received through parenteral or tube feedings in the last 7 days: 0. None; 1. 1% to 25%; 2. 26% to 50%; 3. 51% to 75%; 4. 76% to 100%. b. Code the average fluid intake per day by IV or tube in last 7 days: 0. None; 1. 1 to 500 cc/day; 2. 501 to 1000 cc/day; 3. 1001 to 1500 cc/day; 4. 1501 to 2000 cc/day; 5. 2001 or more cc/day

SECTION L. ORAL/DENTAL STATUS

1.	ORAL STATUS AND DISEASE PREVENTION	Debris (soft, easily movable substances) present in mouth prior to going to bed at night 15 a.; Has dentures or removable bridge b.; Some/all natural teeth lost—does not have or does not use dentures (or partial plates) 15 c.; Broken, loose, or carious teeth 15 d.; Inflamed gums (gingiva); swollen or bleeding gums; oral abscesses; ulcers or rashes 15 e.; Daily cleaning of teeth/dentures or daily mouth care—by resident or staff Not ✓ = 15 f.; *NONE OF ABOVE* g.

SECTION M. SKIN CONDITION

1.	ULCERS (Due to any cause)	*(Record the number of ulcers at each ulcer stage—regardless of cause. If none present at a stage, record "0" (zero). Code all that apply during last 7 days. Code 9 = 9 or more.) [Requires full body exam.]* Number at Stage. a. Stage 1. A persistent area of skin redness (without a break in the skin) that does not disappear when pressure is relieved. b. Stage 2. A partial thickness loss of skin layers that presents clinically as an abrasion, blister, or shallow crater. c. Stage 3. A full thickness of skin is lost, exposing the subcutaneous tissues—presents as a deep crater with or without undermining adjacent tissue. d. Stage 4. A full thickness of skin and subcutaneous tissue is lost, exposing muscle or bone.
2.	TYPE OF ULCER	*(For each type of ulcer, code for the highest stage in the last 7 days using scale in item M1—i.e., 0=none; stages 1, 2, 3, 4)* a. Pressure ulcer—any lesion caused by pressure resulting in damage of underlying tissue 1 = 16; 2, 3, or 4 = 12, 16. b. Stasis ulcer—open lesion caused by poor circulation in the lower extremities
3.	HISTORY OF RESOLVED ULCERS	Resident had an ulcer that was resolved or cured in LAST 90 DAYS 0. No 1. Yes 16
4.	OTHER SKIN PROBLEMS OR LESIONS PRESENT	*(Check all that apply during last 7 days)* Abrasions, bruises a.; Burns (second or third degree) b.; Open lesions other than ulcers, rashes, cuts (e.g., cancer lesions) c.; Rashes—e.g., intertrigo, eczema, drug rash, heat rash, herpes zoster d.; Skin desensitized to pain or pressure 16 e.; Skin tears or cuts (other than surgery) f.; Surgical wounds g.; *NONE OF ABOVE* h.
5.	SKIN TREATMENTS	*(Check all that apply during last 7 days)* Pressure relieving device(s) for chair a.; Pressure relieving device(s) for bed b.; Turning/repositioning program c.; Nutrition or hydration intervention to manage skin problems d.; Ulcer care e.; Surgical wound care f.; Application of dressings (with or without topical medications) other than to feet g.; Application of ointments/medications (other than to feet) h.; Other preventative or protective skin care (other than to feet) i.; *NONE OF ABOVE* j.
6.	FOOT PROBLEMS AND CARE	*(Check all that apply during last 7 days)* Resident has one or more foot problems—e.g., corns, calluses, bunions, hammer toes, overlapping toes, pain, structural problems a.; Infection of the foot—e.g., cellulitis, purulent drainage b.; Open lesions on the foot c.; Nails/calluses trimmed during last 90 days d.; Received preventative or protective foot care (e.g., used special shoes, inserts, pads, toe separators) e.; Application of dressings (with or without topical medications) f.; *NONE OF ABOVE* g.

SECTION N. ACTIVITY PURSUIT PATTERNS

1.	TIME AWAKE (10B only if BOTH N1a = ✓ and N2 = 0)	*(Check appropriate time periods over last 7 days)* Resident awake all or most of time (i.e., naps no more than one hour per time period) in the: Morning 10B a.; Afternoon b.; Evening c.; *NONE OF ABOVE* d.
	(IF RESIDENT IS COMATOSE, SKIP TO SECTION O)	
2.	AVERAGE TIME INVOLVED IN ACTIVITIES	(When awake and not receiving treatments or ADL care) 0. Most—more than 2/3 of time 10B; 1. Some—from 1/3 to 2/3 of time; 2. Little—less than 1/3 of time 10A; 3. None 10A
3.	PREFERRED ACTIVITY SETTINGS	*(Check all settings in which activities are preferred)* Own room a.; Day/activity room b.; Inside NH/off unit c.; Outside facility d.; *NONE OF ABOVE* e.
4.	GENERAL ACTIVITY PREFERENCES (Adapted to resident's current abilities)	*(Check all PREFERENCES whether or not activity is currently available to resident)* Cards/other games a.; Crafts/arts b.; Exercise/sports c.; Music d.; Reading/writing e.; Spiritual/religious activities f.; Trips/shopping g.; Walking/wheeling outdoors h.; Watching TV i.; Gardening or plants j.; Talking or conversing k.; Helping others l.; *NONE OF ABOVE* m.

TRIGGER LEGEND
10A - Activities (Revise)
10B - Activities (Review)
11 - Falls
12 - Nutritional Status
13 - Feeding Tubes
14 - Dehydration/Fluid Maintenance
15 - Dental Care
16 - Pressure Ulcers
17* - Psychotropic Drugs
(*For this to trigger, O4a, b, or c must = 1-7)

MDS 2.0 10/18/94N

Resident ____________________ Numeric Identifier ____________________

5.	PREFERS CHANGE IN DAILY ROUTINE	*Code for resident preferences in daily routines* 0. No change 1. Slight change 2. Major change	
		a. Type of activities in which resident is currently involved 1 or 2 - **10A**	
		b. Extent of resident involvement in activities 1 or 2 - **10A**	

SECTION O. MEDICATIONS

1.	NUMBER OF MEDICATIONS	*(**Record the number of different** medications used in the **last 7 days;** enter "0" if none used)*	
2.	NEW MEDICATIONS	*(Resident currently receiving medications that were initiated during the **last 90 days**)* 0. No 1. Yes	
3.	INJECTIONS	*(**Record the number of DAYS** injections of any type received during the **last 7 days**; enter "0" if none used)*	
4.	DAYS RECEIVED THE FOLLOWING MEDICATION	*(**Record the number of DAYS** during **last 7 days**; enter "0" if not used. Note—enter "1" for long-acting meds used less than weekly)* (NOTE: For **17** to actually be triggered, O4a, b, or c MUST = 1-7 AND at least one additional item marked **17*** must be indicated. See sections B, C, E, G, H, I, J, and K.)	
		a. Antipsychotic 1-7 = **17**	
		b. Antianxiety 1-7 = **11, 17**	
		c. Antidepressant 1-7 = **11, 17**	
		d. Hypnotic	
		e. Diuretic 1-7 = **14**	

SECTION P. SPECIAL TREATMENTS AND PROCEDURES

1. SPECIAL TREATMENTS, PROCEDURES, AND PROGRAMS

a. SPECIAL CARE—*Check treatments received during the **last 14 days*** [Note—count only post admission treatments]

TREATMENTS			
Chemotherapy	a.	Ventilator or respirator	l.
Dialysis	b.	**PROGRAMS**	
IV medication	c.	Alcohol/drug treatment program	m.
Intake/output	d.	Alzheimer's/dementia special care unit	n.
Monitoring acute medical condition	e.	Hospice care	o.
Ostomy care	f.	Pediatric unit	p.
Oxygen therapy	g.	Respite care	q.
Radiation	h.	Training in skills required to return to the community (e.g., taking medications, house work, shopping, transportation, ADLs)	r.
Suctioning	i.	*NONE OF ABOVE*	s.
Tracheostomy care	j.		
Transfusions	k.		

b. THERAPIES—*Record the number of days and total minutes each of the following therapies was administered (for at least 15 minutes a day) in the **last 7 calendar days** (Enter 0 if none or less than 15 min. daily)* [Note—count only post admission therapies]

(A) = # of days administered for 15 minutes or more
(B) = total # of minutes provided in last 7 days

	DAYS (A)	MIN (B)
a. Speech-language pathology and audiology services		
b. Occupational therapy		
c. Physical therapy		
d. Respiratory therapy		
e. Psychological therapy (by any licensed mental health professional)		

2. INTERVENTION PROGRAMS FOR MOOD, BEHAVIOR, COGNITIVE LOSS

(Check all interventions or strategies used in last 7 days—no matter where received)

Special behavior symptom evaluation program	a.
Evaluation by a licensed mental health specialist in last 90 days	b.
Group therapy	c.
Resident-specific deliberate changes in the environment to address mood/behavior patterns—e.g., providing bureau in which to rummage	d.
Reorientation—e.g., cueing	e.
NONE OF ABOVE	f.

3. NURSING REHABILITATION/RESTORATIVE CARE

*Record the **NUMBER OF DAYS** each of the following rehabilitation or restorative techniques or practices was **provided to the resident for more than or equal to 15 minutes** per day in the **last 7 days** (Enter 0 if none or less than 15 min. daily.)*

a. Range of motion (passive)		f. Walking	
b. Range of motion (active)		g. Dressing or grooming	
c. Splint or brace assistance		h. Eating or swallowing	
TRAINING AND SKILL PRACTICE IN:		i. Amputation/prosthesis care	
d. Bed mobility		j. Communication	
e. Transfer		k. Other	

4.	DEVICES AND RESTRAINTS	*(Use the following codes for **last 7 days:**)* 0. Not used 1. Used less than daily 2. Used daily	
		Bed rails	
		a.—Full bed rails on all open sides of bed	
		b.—Other types of side rails used (e.g., half rail, one side)	
		c. Trunk restraint 1 = **11, 18**; 2 = **11, 16, 18**	
		d. Limb restraint 1 or 2 = **18**	
		e. Chair prevents rising 1 or 2 = **18**	
5.	HOSPITAL STAY(S)	Record number of times resident was admitted to hospital with an overnight stay in **last 90 days** (or since last assessment if less than 90 days). *(Enter 0 if no hospital admissions)*	
6.	EMERGENCY ROOM (ER) VISIT(S)	Record number of times resident visited ER without an overnight stay in **last 90 days** (or since last assessment if less than 90 days). *(Enter 0 if no ER visits)*	
7.	PHYSICIAN VISITS	In the **LAST 14 DAYS** (or since admission if less than 14 days in facility) how many days has the physician (or authorized assistant or practitioner) examined the resident? *(Enter 0 if none)*	
8.	PHYSICIAN ORDERS	In the **LAST 14 DAYS** (or since admission if less than 14 days in facility) how many days has the physician (or authorized assistant or practitioner) changed the resident's orders? *Do not include order renewals without change. (Enter 0 if none)*	
9.	ABNORMAL LAB VALUES	Has the resident had any abnormal lab values during the **last 90 days** (or since admission)? 0. No 1. Yes	

SECTION Q. DISCHARGE POTENTIAL AND OVERALL STATUS

1.	DISCHARGE POTENTIAL	a. Resident expresses/indicates preference to return to the community 0. No 1. Yes	
		b. Resident has a support person who is positive toward discharge 0. No 1. Yes	
		c. Stay projected to be of a short duration—discharge projected **within 90 days** (do not include expected discharge due to death) 0. No 1. Within 30 days 2. Within 31-90 days 3. Discharge status uncertain	
2.	OVERALL CHANGE IN CARE NEEDS	Resident's overall self sufficiency has changed significantly as compared to status of **90 days ago** (or since last assessment if less than 90 days) 0. No change 1. Improved—receives fewer supports, needs less restrictive level of care 2. Deteriorated—receives more support	

SECTION R. ASSESSMENT INFORMATION

1.	PARTICIPATION IN ASSESSMENT	a. Resident:	0. No	1. Yes		
		b. Family:	0. No	1. Yes	2. No family	
		c. Significant other:	0. No	1. Yes	2. None	

2. SIGNATURES OF PERSONS COMPLETING THE ASSESSMENT:

a. Signature of RN Assessment Coordinator (sign on above line)

b. Date RN Assessment Coordinator signed as complete ☐☐ — ☐☐ — ☐☐☐☐
Month Day Year

	Title	Sections	Date
c. Other Signatures			Date
d.			Date
e.			Date
f.			Date
g.			Date
h.			Date

TRIGGER LEGEND
10A - Activities (Revise)
11 - Falls
14 - Dehydration/Fluid Maintenance
16 - Pressure Ulcers
17 - Psychotropic Drugs
18 - Physical Restraints

7 of 8

MDS 2.0 10/18/94N

SECTION V. RESIDENT ASSESSMENT PROTOCOL SUMMARY Numeric Identifier________

Resident's Name:	Medical Record No.:

1. Check if RAP is triggered.
2. For each triggered RAP, use the RAP guidelines to identify areas needing further assessment. Document relevant assessment information regarding the resident's status.
   - Describe:
     - —Nature of the condition (may include presence or lack of objective data and subjective complaints).
     - —Complications and risk factors that affect your decision to proceed to care planning.
     - —Factors that must be considered in developing individualized care plan interventions.
     - —Need for referrals/further evaluation by appropriate health professionals.
   - Documentation should support your decision-making regarding whether to proceed with a care plan for a triggered RAP and the type(s) of care plan interventions that are appropriate for a particular resident.
   - Documentation may appear anywhere in the clinical record (e.g., progress notes, consults, flowsheets, etc.).
3. Indicate under the Location of RAP Assessment Documentation column where information related to the RAP assessment can be found.
4. For each triggered RAP, indicate whether a new care plan, care plan revision, or continuation of current care plan is necessary to address the problem(s) identified in your assessment. The Care Planning Decision column must be completed within 7 days of completing the RAI (MDS and RAPs).

A. RAP Problem Area	(a) Check if Triggered	Location and Date of RAP Assessment Documentation	(b) Care Planning Decision—check if addressed in care plan
1. DELIRIUM			
2. COGNITIVE LOSS			
3. VISUAL FUNCTION			
4. COMMUNICATION			
5. ADL FUNCTIONAL/ REHABILITATION POTENTIAL			
6. URINARY INCONTINENCE AND INDWELLING CATHETER			
7. PSYCHOSOCIAL WELL-BEING			
8. MOOD STATE			
9. BEHAVIORAL SYMPTOMS			
10. ACTIVITIES			
11. FALLS			
12. NUTRITIONAL STATUS			
13. FEEDING TUBES			
14. DEHYDRATION/FLUID MAINTENANCE			
15. ORAL/DENTAL CARE			
16. PRESSURE ULCERS			
17. PSYCHOTROPIC DRUG USE			
18. PHYSICAL RESTRAINTS			

B. ____ 2. ☐☐–☐☐–☐☐☐☐ (Month Day Year)

1. Signature of RN Coordinator for RAP Assessment Process

____ 4. ☐☐–☐☐–☐☐☐☐ (Month Day Year)

3. Signature of Person Completing Care Planning Decision

Form 39728L

8 of 8

MDS 2.0 10/18/94N

Glossary

ADL—activities of daily living which include eating, toileting, dressing, bathing, grooming, and mobility.

Age Appropriate—a normalized activity or piece of equipment that is suitable and respectful of the age of the person involved.

Bilateral—using both sides of the body together.

Dementia Syndrome—a group of symptoms which negatively influence cognitive performance and memory. There are over 70 causes, some of which are reversible. The most common form of dementia is Alzheimer's disease.

Flow—a peak leisure experience.

Function—what people are capable of doing in their own environment.

Geriatrics—medical practice and treatment of older adults.

Gerontology—the multidisciplinary study of aging.

IADL—instrumental activities of daily living which include money management, household chores, use of transportation, shopping, health maintenance, communication, and safety preparedness.

Leisure—a state of mind that results from voluntary interactions with oneself, others, or the environment.

Older Adult—a individual who is over 65 years of age.

Old-Old—those individuals over 75 years of age.

Perceived Freedom—feeling resulting from freely choosing leisure.

Proprioception—sensing movement, bending, and location of parts of the body.

Range of Motion—range of motion or flexibility.

Sensory Integration—neurophysiological process by which sensory information is organized and interpreted.

Young-Old—65-75 years of age.

Subject Index

Other Books From Venture Publishing, Inc.

The A•B•Cs of Behavior Change: Skills for Working with Behavior Problems in Nursing Homes
by Margaret D. Cohn, Michael A. Smyer and Ann L. Horgas
Activity Experiences and Programming Within Long-Term Care
by Ted Tedrick and Elaine R. Green
The Activity Gourmet
by Peggy Powers
Advanced Concepts for Geriatric Nursing Assistants
by Carolyn A. McDonald
Adventure Education
edited by John C. Miles and Simon Priest
Assessment: The Cornerstone of Activity Programs
by Ruth Perschbacher
At-Risk Youth and Gangs—A Resource Manual for the Parks and Recreation Professional—Expanded and Updated
by The California Park and Recreation Society
Behavior Modification in Therapeutic Recreation: An Introductory Learning Manual
by John Dattilo and William D. Murphy
Benefits of Leisure
edited by B. L. Driver, Perry J. Brown and George L. Peterson
Benefits of Recreation Research Update
by Judy M. Sefton and W. Kerry Mummery
Beyond Bingo: Innovative Programs for the New Senior
by Sal Arrigo, Jr., Ann Lewis and Hank Mattimore
The Community Tourism Industry Imperative—The Necessity, The Opportunities, Its Potential
by Uel Blank
Dimensions of Choice: A Qualitative Approach to Recreation, Parks, and Leisure Research
by Karla A. Henderson
Evaluating Leisure Services: Making Enlightened Decisions
by Karla A. Henderson with M. Deborah Bialeschki
Evaluation of Therapeutic Recreation Through Quality Assurance
edited by Bob Riley
The Evolution of Leisure: Historical and Philosophical Perspectives—Second Printing
by Thomas Goodale and Geoffrey Godbey
The Game Finder—A Leader's Guide to Great Activities
by Annette C. Moore
Great Special Events and Activities
by Annie Morton, Angie Prosser and Sue Spangler
Inclusive Leisure Services: Responding to the Rights of People with Disabilities
by John Dattilo
Internships in Recreation and Leisure Services: A Practical Guide for Students
by Edward E. Seagle, Jr., Ralph W. Smith and Lola M. Dalton
Interpretation of Cultural and Natural Resources
by Douglas M. Knudson, Ted T. Cable and Larry Beck

Introduction to Leisure Services—7th Edition
by H. Douglas Sessoms and Karla A. Henderson
Leadership and Administration of Outdoor Pursuits, Second Edition
by Phyllis Ford and James Blanchard
Leisure And Family Fun (LAFF)
by Mary Atteberry-Rogers
The Leisure Diagnostic Battery: Users Manual and Sample Forms
by Peter A. Witt and Gary Ellis
Leisure Diagnostic Battery Computer Software
by Gary Ellis and Peter A. Witt
Leisure Education: A Manual of Activities and Resources
by Norma J. Stumbo and Steven R. Thompson
Leisure Education II: More Activities and Resources
by Norma J. Stumbo
Leisure Education: Program Materials for Persons with Developmental Disabilities
by Kenneth F. Joswiak
Leisure Education Program Planning: A Systematic Approach
by John Dattilo and William D. Murphy
Leisure in Your Life: An Exploration, Fourth Edition
by Geoffrey Godbey
A Leisure of One's Own: A Feminist Perspective on Women's Leisure
by Karla Henderson, M. Deborah Bialeschki, Susan M. Shaw and Valeria J. Freysinger
Leisure Services in Canada: An Introduction
by Mark S. Searle and Russell E. Brayley
Leveraging the Benefits of Parks and Recreation: The Phoenix Project
by The California Park and Recreation Society
Marketing for Parks, Recreation, and Leisure
by Ellen L. O'Sullivan
Outdoor Recreation Management: Theory and Application, Third Edition
by Alan Jubenville and Ben Twight
Planning Parks for People
by John Hultsman, Richard L. Cottrell and Wendy Zales Hultsman
Private and Commercial Recreation
edited by Arlin Epperson
The Process of Recreation Programming Theory and Technique, Third Edition
by Patricia Farrell and Herberta M. Lundegren
Protocols for Recreation Therapy Programs
edited by Jill Kelland, along with the Recreation Therapy Staff at Alberta Hospital—Edmonton
Quality Management: Applications for Therapeutic Recreation
edited by Bob Riley
Recreation and Leisure: Issues in an Era of Change, Third Edition
edited by Thomas Goodale and Peter A. Witt
The Recreation Connection to Self-Esteem—A Resource Manual for the Park, Recreation and Community Services Professional
by The California Park and Recreation Society

Other Books From Venture Publishing, Inc.

Recreation Economic Decisions: Comparing Benefits and Costs
by Richard G. Walsh
Recreation Programming and Activities for Older Adults
by Jerold E. Elliott and Judith A. Sorg-Elliott
Reference Manual for Writing Rehabilitation Therapy Treatment Plans
by Penny Hogberg and Mary Johnson
Research in Therapeutic Recreation: Concepts and Methods
edited by Marjorie J. Malkin and Christine Z. Howe
Risk Management in Therapeutic Recreation: A Component of Quality Assurance
by Judith Voelkl
A Social History of Leisure Since 1600
by Gary Cross
The Sociology of Leisure
by John R. Kelly and Geoffrey Godbey
A Study Guide for National Certification in Therapeutic Recreation
by Gerald O'Morrow and Ron Reynolds
Therapeutic Recreation: Cases and Exercises
by Barbara C. Wilhite and M. Jean Keller
Therapeutic Recreation Protocol for Treatment of Substance Addictions
by Rozanne W. Faulkner
A Training Manual for Americans With Disabilities Act Compliance in Parks and Recreation Settings
by Carol Stensrud
Understanding Leisure and Recreation: Mapping the Past, Charting the Future
edited by Edgar L. Jackson and Thomas L. Burton

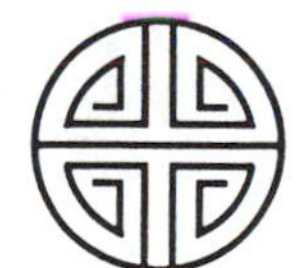

Venture Publishing
1999 Cato Avenu
State College, PA 1

Phone: (814) 234-4561; FAX